Birth Ambassadors

Doulas and the Re-Emergence of Woman-Supported Birth

Christine H. Morton, Ph.D.
with Elayne G. Clift, M.A.

Foreword by Holly Kennedy, Ph.D., CNM
Afterword by Mark Sloan, MD

Photographs by
Kyndal May, MFA, CD(DONA), BDT(DONA), LCCE &
Vuefinder Photography | San Diego Birth Photographer

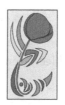

Praeclarus Press, LLC
©2014 Christine Morton and Elayne Clift. All rights reserved
www.PraeclarusPress.com

Praeclarus Press, LLC

2504 Sweetgum Lane

Amarillo, Texas 79124 USA

806-367-9950

www.PraeclarusPress.com

DISCLAIMER

The information contained in this publication is advisory only and is not intended to replace sound clinical judgment or individualized patient care. The author disclaims all warranties, whether expressed or implied, including any warranty as the quality, accuracy, safety, or suitability of this information for any particular purpose.

ISBN: 978-1-939807-06-9

Cover Design: Ken Tackett

Acquisition & Development: Kathleen Kendall-Tackett

Copy Editing: Diana Cassar-Uhl

Layout & Design: Todd Rollison

Operations: Scott Sherwood

Table of Contents

Index of Photos

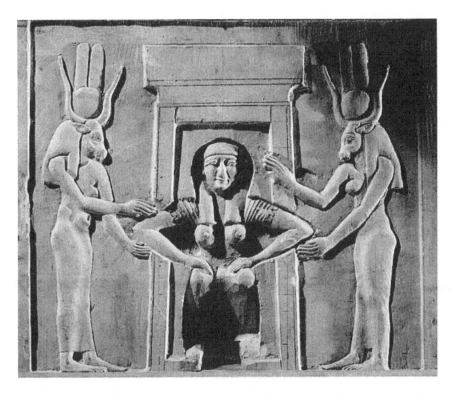

Photo 1: A relief from the temple of Hathor at Dendera. A squatting woman is giving birth assisted by two goddesses. Egypt. Ptolemaic Period c.323-30 BC.
Credit Line: Werner Forman Archive/ Egyptian Museum, Cairo. Used with permission.

Acknowledgements

Christine Morton

I first thank all the doulas in my life and in this study who shared their experiences with me. With this project, I strive to honor all those who work to improve maternity care and outcomes.

Heartfelt gratitude goes to my life partner, Marc Smith, and our children Eli and Madeline, who each, in their own unique way, encouraged me to "just finish the book." Marc's unwavering support and love has been a treasured gift. I appreciate his patience and willingness to listen to me talk (and talk some more) about doulas and birth. His sociological insights have been helpful as well! I also thank my parents Ken and Mary Morton, my sisters Joanne Morton and Jennifer Morton, and my in-laws, Diane Smith and Ron Bohr, for their faith in me and for their support along my journey.

Several dear friends and colleagues have given me intellectual support and helpful suggestions over the years. Thank you to Debra Bingham, Jennifer Block, Carole Browner, Valerie Cape, Raymond DeVries, Nicole Heidbreder, Walker Karraa, Maggie Kusenbach, Paula Lantz, Judy Lothian, Lisa Kane Low, Theresa Morris, Adina Nack, Theta Pavis, Debra Pascali-Bonaro, Katie Pine, Kerreen Reiger, Amy Romano, Sharon Storton, my CMQCC colleagues, the Maternity Support Survey team and all the ReproNetworkers. Thanks to research assistant, Sheeva Hariri, who conducted several interviews with Los Angeles doulas. During the course of my dissertation research, my open-minded committee members Carole Browner, John Heritage, Laura Gómez, and the late Melvin Pollner believed in this project, and me, and for that I am grateful. A very special thank you to Robbie Davis-Floyd, whose words of encouragement during a difficult transition helped me redirect my journey toward doulas and follow my passion, and for her thoughtful critique and sustained enthusiasm for this project even as it lay gestating for some time.

The Pacific Association for Labor Support Board of Directors whole-heartedly supported me professionally and personally and taught me so many things during my time in Seattle. Members of the DONA International board of directors answered lots of emails with grace. Thanks to Natasha Giddings for providing a crucial piece to labor support history. I couldn't have done it without contributions from Penny Simkin, Jan Dowers, Polly Perez, Henci Goer, Robin Elise Weiss, Dr. John Kennell, Dr. Marshall Klaus, Debbie Young, Sharon Ledbetter, Tracy Peters, Kristin Minor, Jessica Porter, Suzanne Arms, Joan Barbour, Claudia Lowe, and Pamela Eakins, PhD, all of whom generously gave their time and attention to my requests for information and materials about doula history. Penny Simkin, in particular, led by example and offered me key advice during one conversation that has stuck with me ever since, encouraging me to think how to make the most impact with this project. I am indebted to her for helping me understand there is a world and an audience for my insights outside academia.

I am grateful for Kathleen Kendall-Tackett and Praeclarus Press for their support and enthusiasm for this book. Thank you to our contributors who wrote wonderful personal stories. Thank you to Holly Kennedy and Mark Sloan for your support and contributions. The photos from Kyndal May and Catie Stephens have immeasurably enhanced this book's appeal and show the power and care embodied in labor support in ways that words cannot. And most of all, I'm grateful to Elayne Clift, whose call for doula narratives piqued my interest and then opened a door for a wonderfully synchronous project of stories and analysis. Her enthusiasm and praise for my dissertation helped me find the confidence to do the hard labor of birthing this book, through multiple revisions and a much longer time line than we originally expected. I wouldn't have done it at all, or as well, without you. Every author needs a doula, and I found mine in Elayne. Thank you from the bottom of my heart.

Elayne Clift

To those whom Christine has cited, I add my own gratitude. I also offer heartfelt thanks to all those people who responded to my call for contributions by sharing their personal stories—there were many more than we could include and all of them were equally compelling. These contributions enhanced the outcome of this book immeasurably.

I am grateful to Holly Kennedy and Mark Sloan for their Foreword and Afterword, which form such rich "bookends" to this work.

For my husband, Arnold, who so often cooks so that I can compose; for my daughter, Rachel, who champions my work and already has a huge audience lined up for this book; and for my son, David, who just loves to brag about his mom, my deep and abiding love.

And for Christine, literary partner and new friend par excellence—no other collaboration I can imagine could be as joyful. Thank you for "getting it," doing it, and sharing it.

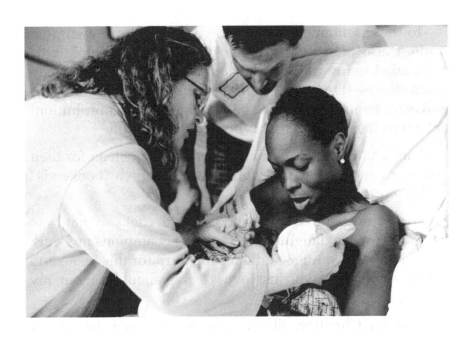

Photo 2: Doula helps new mother with breastfeeding latch as new father looks on.
Photo by Vuefinder Photography | San Diego Birth Photographer.

Preface
by Elayne Clift

I'm a baby freak, plain and simple. As a young candy strip-er I routinely snuck into the pediatric ward so I could rock sick kids. While my high school friends dated, I babysat. If I hadn't been a product of the fifties, I might have considered becoming an obstetrician or a midwife. Instead I followed the path that most girls my age did: I went to college for a liberal arts degree and then became a secretary—a medical secretary.

My real career began when I became program director in 1979 for the National Women's Health Network, a Washington, D.C.-based education and advocacy organization dedicated to humane, holistic, evidence-based, feminist approaches to women's healthcare. In 1985, I went to Nairobi for the final international conference of the United Nations Decade for Women (1975-1985). Inspired by that amazing event and armed with a master's degree in health communication, I began working internationally on behalf of women and children, always trying to bring a gender lens to the table.

In the midst of all this, I gave birth twice. My children were born in the 1970s as the women's health movement, and individual women, were beginning to advocate for natural childbirth and to resist the traumas of overly medicalized birth experiences. We took Lamaze classes, learned about breast-feeding, and expected dads to be active in our deliveries. I was lucky: not only were my labors quick and unremarkable, the small community hospital where I delivered was sympathetic to the changes taking place in birthing. There were no monitors, no drugs "to take the edge off" if you didn't want them, no enemas, no shaving, and no macho-docs (although I couldn't talk my doctor out of the episiotomy). I labored with my nurse and my husband, and when the time came to push,

I watched my babies come into this world in total awe of what had just happened and what I had done.

Several years ago, I learned that my local hospital had a volunteer doula program. Signing up was a no-brainer, and I've now had the honor of supporting many women and their partners as they've done the hard work of delivering a baby. I've even had the opportunity to be a "birth ambassador" to women in Somaliland. Not one of the women I served has failed to tell me afterwards, "I couldn't have done it without you!"

One of the early births I attended stands out in my mind. It was a first pregnancy, and the woman labored stoically for 36 hours, pushing for five, before her son was born. As the hours passed, I held her hand, wet her lips, wiped strands of matted hair from her eyes, and rubbed her back. "You can do this," I whispered in her ear when she grew doubtful. "You're doing a magnificent job! Soon your baby will be born." As the baby finally crowned, wet, dark hair pressing urgently against her, I held the mother's leg in my arm, her hand clenching my free wrist as she cried out with that guttural groan of a woman pushing her child to life outside the womb. And suddenly, there he was, head between her legs, wet and pinking up even as his perfect little body, full of blood and mucus swam into being. Later, swaddled and suckling at his mother's breast, his father, eyes wet, whispered across the bed to me, "Women's bodies are so miraculous." "Yes," I said, my own eyes filling, "Miraculous." Always miraculous, no matter how many times you give witness to a woman giving birth.

That is why I feel privileged to do this voluntary work, and why I felt compelled to do this book. It is simply an honor to give witness to birth, and to offer as many women as possible the opportunity to have a birth that is supported, memorable, and full of joy.

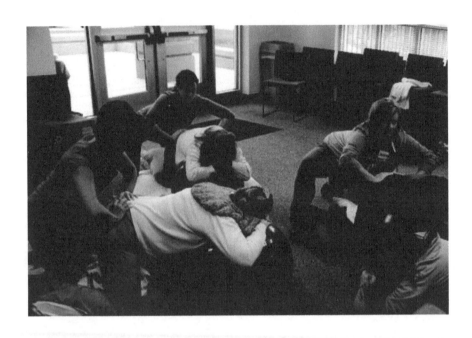

Photo 3. Doulas-in-training practicing double hip squeeze, a labor support comfort measure, on each other.
Photo by Kyndal May.

Foreword
Holly Powell Kennedy, Ph.D., CNM, FACNM, FAAN

According to the *Oxford English Dictionary*, an ambassador is "an official messenger; an envoy ... to perform special duties."[1] It is an apt description of the doula, who works to guide women in the foreign land of hospital labor and birth. I speak specifically to the hospital birth setting because this is where we have really lost our way in the United States birthing nation.

Over one third of women in the United States will have a surgical birth and almost half will have their labors medically induced. Few women give birth experiencing the power of endogenous endorphins, in a position they choose, nourished, or fully supported by someone they know and trust throughout the process. Only ten percent will have a midwife attend their birth, a standard in many countries with outcomes far better than the United States, which resides among the bottom tier of developed countries in infant mortality.

The mantra of United States medicine is "evidence-based practice," yet care practices known to support women's physiologic capacity to birth are largely ignored, and we do not focus on broad goals of preparing a healthy mother and family. Reasons for this disregard are complex, but are culturally reflective of education and media exposures, a fearful and risk-aversive society, and trust in technology rather than in the power of women's bodies.

Christine Morton and Elayne Clift have unlocked a window into the current world of childbearing, and the role of the doula in that arena. The scenario is far different from the

---

1 *Oxford English Dictionary*. (2010). Ambassador. Retrieved December 20, 2010. Available at: http://oed.com/view/Entry/6095?redirectedFrom=ambassador#.

1960s, when women struggled to get fathers into the labor room. Now, families are welcome, but the ability of a woman to influence what she can do in that room is essentially limited in many hospitals. Every woman wants to do her best for her baby as she travels the journey to motherhood. However, insuring her ability to obtain care that capitalizes on evidence-based practices is challenged. Her ability to advocate for herself in the height of labor can be daunting; hence the need for a doula.

Doula attended birth is not a return to the "good old days" when women were surrounded by neighbors of varying competency. Rather, it represents an evolution to an educated, supportive companion who knows how to support the childbearing process and advocate for the woman if needed. The doula is the envoy to provide a message to all present of a commitment to meeting the woman's needs and desires for her birth.

Some clinicians (midwives, nurses, physicians) will be threatened by the doula. I would encourage them to turn threat into opportunity. Remember the triad of evidence-based care: a) scientific evidence, b) clinician expertise, and c) the desires of the woman. Sit down and talk with the woman, her family, and the doula about what they are hoping to experience. Involve everyone who will be working to care for the woman in the birth. An environment of trust will be established, and fear will be turned to confidence for both woman and clinician. To truly place a woman at the center of care and to facilitate her innate capacity to bear a child without medical intervention requires commitment to thinking differently about birth and power. This attitude shift is essential if every woman is going to have the chance for the very best care possible that is associated with best outcomes. This book provides an articulate and thoughtful exploration of the issues facing us in child-bearing care today with the doula providing a much-needed voice in the debate.

Holly Powell Kennedy, Ph.D., CNM, FACNM, FAAN, Varney Professor of Midwifery at Yale University and Past-President of the American College of Nurse-Midwives (ACNM)

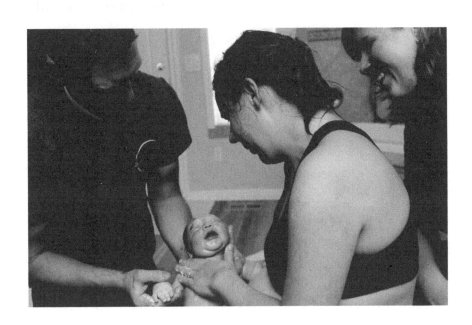

Photo 4. New parents greet their just-born baby as doula looks on.
Photo by Kyndal May.

Personal Story

THE BEST BEGINNING
Emme Dague Amble

When I heard the word "doula," I reacted the same way most people do when they first hear this strange word: "What's a doula?" I asked quizzically. I truly believe that the answer to this question was life-changing for our family.

When I found out I was pregnant with our first child, I was filled with joy, amazement, and wonder. Very soon, however, I was filled with questions. What should I expect throughout the pregnancy? How would I care for our sweet babe when he or she made his or her arrival? Childbirth itself was a total unknown. I dove into the world of pregnancy and childbirth research eagerly, and soon found myself in a maze of various and conflicting philosophies, facts, and opinions, voiced by people who called themselves experts, all of them sure theirs was the "correct" way to give birth. If I chose "their" way, it seemed to be an almost-guaranteed running start on a happy, healthy childhood and parent-child relationship. How was I to know if I was on the right track? What if I made the wrong choice? What if something went wrong?

I certainly wanted a healthy baby, but as I read more and began to form my own opinions, I realized that I also wanted to experience childbirth as a rite of passage, as a way for my husband and me to connect, both to each other and to the baby about to join us on our journey. I wanted to feel supported and safe, that my choices would be respected even if they varied from the standard operating procedure of the hospital. Of course, I had chosen caregivers whom I could trust to give me a high standard of care. I knew they only wanted a safe and healthy outcome for both mother and child, but I knew I wanted something more. More personal? More home-like? I wasn't sure exactly what it was, or how to make it happen.

I continued to devour every childbirth preparation book I could get my hands on, and signed up for the childbirth preparation series at our hospital. I knew that preparation would be a key piece to the puzzle for the birth I was hoping for. I thought that the more we knew, and the more we practiced the breathing and comfort techniques, and the more my husband knew about the process, the better. Soon, however, I could see that my husband's enthusiasm for childbirth information just wasn't the same as mine! He loved me and was happy the baby was on its way, but the "hee-hee-hoo's" of the breathing exercises, the counting, the guided imagery, left him giggling at best, and caused his eyelids to droop at worst. My husband was going to be a wonderful emotional comfort to me at the birth, but he wasn't going to be the advocate and knowledgeable birth partner I knew I would need.

A few weeks into our class series, our instructor revealed that she was a doula. She explained that her job would be to come alongside us during labor, to soothe and comfort physically and emotionally, and to support our choices in this amazing moment of our life together. It was an Aha! moment for me. Yes! This was the missing piece! A knowledgeable woman, who had "gone before" in her knowledge of the birth process, as well as the comfort measures, hospital procedures, and the emotional needs of both of us. This was perfect. At first my husband was skeptical, even offended a little, to think that I might need someone other than him to feel safe and supported at our child's birth. But as we talked more, she gently explained that she in no way takes the place of the father. In fact, her presence often freed the father up to be more emotionally available to the mother, since he didn't have to worry about knowing all the specifics of comfort measures, or even the stages of the birth process. My husband was relieved to know he would be free to just love on me in his own way, and he also loved that he wouldn't be the only set of hands if (when) I needed a very long back rub. Even the simple freedom of knowing there would be someone on deck in case of a long labor, allowing him to take a quick nap or go grab a bite to eat, made the presence of a doula even more enticing to him.

It was also comforting to me to know that she would be a sounding board for questions that may come up when presented with various medical interventions as the labor progressed. She said that she would in no way interfere with our caregivers' procedures, but that she would be available to answer questions about the risks and benefits of each one, helping us to make informed choices along the way if our birth did not go as planned.

As our due date approached, we diligently followed through with our class series, made our birth plan, and felt confident going into our labor that we would have a wonderful, "easy" natural birth. With our doula at our side, we felt that everything would be smooth sailing. We had chosen to have a midwife-attended hospital birth, and were confident that we had put together a wonderful plan.

What I didn't plan for was to go into labor at 37 weeks. Technically safe to go ahead with labor, I wasn't worried and was even a little relieved when my water broke during an afternoon nap almost three weeks early. However, after nearly fifteen hours with no contractions, my caregivers were starting to get worried. The baby needed to be born within 24 hours of the water breaking, and I wasn't getting anywhere. Our doula helped us to make a choice to go ahead with a prostaglandin gel induction in hopes that it would give us a kick start to our labor, preserving our desire to have as few interventions as possible. At that time (and without my knowledge), they also gave me a dose of Cytotec, now proven to carry the risk of causing dangerously strong contractions.

At first, the labor began normally, and our doula gently encouraged us with various comfort measures, and we enjoyed casually laughing and chatting with her between contractions. In a few hours, however, I found myself in a futile attempt to manage contractions with double and triple peaks of pain lasting longer than two minutes with little to no break in between. I had gotten into the tub earlier in labor hoping to find some relief, but now I found myself panicking, unable to get ahead of the pain, with my husband also in an emotional panic wondering if something was seriously wrong. In addition, this was all happening during a shift change in hospital staff. I remember being aware of a crowd of people at the door of the bathroom looking at me with sympathy, as they tried to explain to the next group of staff what was going on. My midwife could barely squeeze by to get her fetoscope down to my belly to check on the baby. My husband shrank back into the corner to make room for all the staff to get by. Tears were streaming down his cheeks. I felt completely alone, out of control, terrified.

At that moment, my doula absolutely saved me. She swooped in close, allowing the midwife to do all her work, and called to me in a firm yet gentle voice. Her voice penetrated all the chaos that surrounded me outside and within, and got my attention. "Open your eyes!" she gently commanded. I was unable to respond, so again she said, "Open your eyes!" My eyes met hers, and she stayed with me, counting loudly over the din of the staff's discussion of my progress, "Count with me!" she said. Feebly, I followed her lead, anything to get myself into a rhythm, and my mind off the seemingly unbearable pain. My husband was able to come back in close, hold my hand knowing that someone else was helping me, in a way the midwife simply couldn't given her medical duties. His panic melted away, knowing I was being taken care of. The hospital staff was able to settle into their own routines, sensing the energy of the room changing from frantic to a more settled, though admittedly intense rhythm. Her firm, yet gentle coaching helped all of us, including the hospital staff, to settle down, and get back to doing the work at hand.

My doula did her job of caring for my physical need for comfort, focus, and rhythm, which freed my husband up to simply love me with his voice, to hold my hand. In turn, my midwife and nursing team could then do what they do best, to care for my medical needs, and making sure baby was safe. My pain level was still high, but my doula's voice helped me to gain control, and work with the contractions instead of letting the pain take over and push me into panic mode, which inevitably would have dangerously prolonged my labor. After one hour of pushing, I delivered a healthy baby girl, almost exactly 24 hours after my water had broken. Just in time.

The presence of our doula made all the difference, and I believed helped us avoid many medical interventions, perhaps even a c-section had my labor stalled or become truly unbearable due to the heightened pain I experienced from the Cytotec-induced contractions.

A few days after our return home, our doula gave us another amazing gift. She had been taking notes throughout the labor, and had typed up our birth story, recording many tender moments between my husband and me, words whispered by my love that I had already forgotten. She preserved the beautiful moments of our birth story for us, when otherwise they would have been lost to me forever. Our story became even sweeter with this piece of our history being written down for us. Our doula helped us in so many ways. By helping us to make informed choices, coming in close and "taking charge" when the labor got too big for us, and allowing our caregivers to do their best work, we achieved the best possible outcome. Happy mama, healthy baby, relieved papa. We were off to our very best beginning.

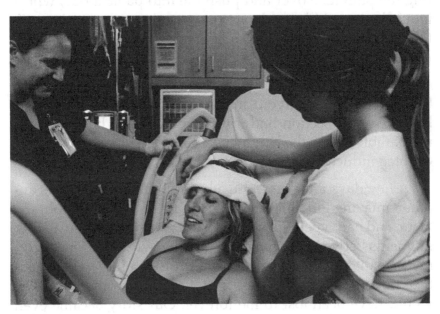

Photo 5. Doula applies cool cloth to laboring woman's head with nurse alongside.
Photo by Kyndal May.

Introduction

When the word "doula" comes up in a conversation about childbirth, there are two typical responses: "What's that, like a midwife?" or "Oh! I had a doula!" The first response reveals how little is known in many quarters about the resurgence of a longstanding tradition—women supporting other birthing women—now taking place within modern birth settings. The latter exclamation is often a grateful acknowledgement of the support she received from her doula in the form of information, physical comfort, and emotional reassurance during labor and birth.

More women of childbearing age have become aware of doulas and their role, and there is renewed interest in the social history and politics of childbirth practices in the United States, as evidenced in popular documentaries, such as *The Business of Being Born*, and books about the history of birth (Cassidy, 2006; Epstein, 2010). We have seen an explosion of entertainment media focusing on celebrity pregnancies, with daily updates on reality TV personalities' latest food and clothing choices, and daddy dramas while pregnant. There was even a film released in 2012 based on the bestselling childbirth advice book, What to Expect When You're Expecting. However, entertainment media show a narrow view of cultural and medical practices, and this view typically reflects a dominant social understanding of pregnancy and childbirth: that it is risky, dangerous, and requires routine medical intervention. We see this in plot lines where women experience one labor contraction and are rushed to the hospital immediately, and only the heroic efforts of medical personnel save the mother or the baby from catastrophe.

Doulas are still minor actors in the public drama of entertainment pregnancies, yet they are emerging in everyday pregnancies—doulas attended 6% of births in the U.S. in 2012, and increasingly appear in stories and research about improving birth outcomes. Doulas engage both popular stories and medical science; they are eagerly interested in minutiae of personal birth experiences, but decry what they see as simplified and misinformed birth stories in the public sphere. Doulas wade into cultural narratives that claim birth is a dangerous, risky time, best managed by medical experts. They articulate an alternative perspective, also known as the midwifery model, that says birth is a usually a normal physiological process, and in that case, best handled by midwives or other low-intervention providers. Doulas base their claims for this alternative perspective on science and experience.

In this book, we show how doulas have entered the debates around birth in the United States. Doulas, or, as we call them, "birth ambassadors," translate and cross the borders between media portrayals, mainstream medical practices, and the midwifery model of birth, articulating a message that is often drowned out by those with greater access to larger marketing budgets. As birth ambassadors, doulas offer to personally accompany women and their families through a strange, yet familiar landscape: the world of hospital-based childbirth.

Birth was once a mysterious, little-talked-about experience, accessible only through formal childbirth education classes where expectant couples watched a film or video showing hospital-based practices and graphic depictions of childbirth. Today, birth stories can be read on the Internet and in books, or viewed on YouTube and reality TV shows. A mere 40 years ago, most American fathers were not present at their child's birth. Today, a birthing woman is encouraged to bring not only the father of the baby, but her family, friends, and co-workers are accommodated, if not actively welcomed at hospital maternity wards. A pregnant woman's doula is also welcome, and in some hospitals, doulas are included in a hospital-based volunteer program, available to women who request or have need of this type of labor support.

This book tells the story of how doulas emerged in maternity care in the United States, explores the science behind claims of the effectiveness of continuous labor support, and offers an examination of the contradictions and accomplishments doulas experience as they do their work. It combines the results of a sociological research study on the history and experiences of doulas in the United States by Christine Morton with personal narratives from women who have worked as doulas, or had a doula at their births, collected and edited by Elayne Clift. The juxtaposition of the narratives with the chapters featuring Morton's analysis of the history and nature of doula practice provides a fuller picture of what motivates doulas, the nature of their work, and the challenges and dilemmas that doulas and their organizations face in their quest to become ambassadors to the world of birth for pregnant women and their families.

What are Doulas?

Doulas are birthing companions trained to provide continuous, one-on-one care and physical, emotional, and informational support to women and their partners throughout labor and childbirth. The doula role and definition have changed over time. The word doula comes from the Greek, and refers to a woman who personally serves another woman. In 1977, anthropologist Dana Raphael adopted this term to refer to experienced mothers who assisted new mothers in breastfeeding and newborn care in the Philippines. This definition centers around a community practice in postpartum, and is still used to refer to postpartum doulas, who help new mothers at home with emotional support and encouragement, light housekeeping, meal preparation, care for other children, and information about breastfeeding and other newborn activities (Placksin, 1994; Webber, 2012).

Around the same time, physician-researchers Marshall Klaus and John Kennell were conducting what would become the first of several randomized clinical trials on the medical outcomes of doula-attended births. Klaus and Kennell adopted the term "doula" to refer to women who provide supportive care during labor and childbirth, as well as those who provide postpartum support, and published their first study in 1980. Since then, the efficacy and impact of continuous labor support has been shown by several research studies to positively affect childbirth outcomes. One of the paradoxes this book will address is how doulas can affect birth outcomes since, unlike midwives and nurses, doulas receive no clinical training, and have no direct responsibility for the health and medical well-being of the pregnant woman or the newborn.

Although the community practice of supporting women through birth and postpartum is as ancient as human society, the role of the doula was formally conceived at The Birth Place in Menlo Park, California, a freestanding birth center licensed by the state in 1979. The founders of The Birth Place were aware of the research described above, and designed the doula, initially referred to as a childbirth assistant, as a central component of the birth center (Eakins, 1984). Childbirth assistants provided labor support and early breastfeeding assistance, as well as meals, to new mothers and their families. They also did the laundry and physical cleanup of the facility after the birth. The first doula training in the U.S. was held at The Birth Place in 1985. Five major national organizations, as well as several regional organizations, now offer training and certification programs, in addition to continuing education and referral services. There are no official statistics on how many doulas are in practice, but the largest of the organizations, DONA International, reports 6,154 members and over 8,500 certified doulas in 2012.[1]

---

1 http://www.dona.org/aboutus/statistics.php, accessed 5/11/13.

Doula Training and Practice Models

The most typical training model is a four-day labor support workshop that combines reading assignments, didactic lectures, and hands-on exercises. In these workshops, aspiring doulas learn basic childbirth physiology and standard medical management of childbirth. They also receive an introduction to the midwifery model of birth and are introduced to scientific research literature on birth practices. The main focus in doula training is a particular set of goals: " ... to support and nurture the laboring woman physically and emotionally, to provide information and advocacy and to protect the memory of her birth experience" (DONA International, www. dona.org).[2]

There are a number of models for labor support doulas, including independent, volunteer, and community-based practice models. Each model may envision and structure the doula's role differently. Many independent-practice doulas meet their clients once or twice prenatally to discuss the woman's birth plan and the doula's role. The doula may have additional telephone or email contact before being called to join her client in labor, either at her home or at the birth site. The doula then stays continuously with the laboring woman until the baby is born and the new family has settled down to rest. Doulas next meet their clients anywhere between two and six weeks postpartum to review the birth, offer referrals for additional support if needed, receive final payment for their services (if they are not volunteers), and end their official relationship. Volunteer doulas may or may not meet their clients in advance.

---

2 Although several organizations train and certify doulas, this analysis will refer most centrally to DONA International's definition of the doula role and scope of work. The organization was formed in 1992 as Doulas of North America, but changed its name in 2004 to DONA International. This book refers to the organization as either term, or just DONA, depending on the context.

In some models, labor and delivery nurses notify volunteer doulas when a woman is admitted to the hospital. Community-based doulas may have extensive prenatal and postpartum contact with their clients, similar to a caseworker model. A growing number of doulas work as employees and/or volunteers in hospital-based and/or community-based doula programs in the U.S. The majority of doulas, however, work as independent practitioners, hired directly by the pregnant woman for a fee ranging on average between $400 and $1,000, depending on the region of the country.[3] Many doulas offer sliding-scale fees or will accept barter arrangements.

The Doula Role in Modern Maternity Care

Doulas occupy a unique outsider-within role in modern maternity care. Having carved out women's emotional, physical, and informational needs during childbirth as their specialized domain, the presence of doulas is both a critique of the current system for not being centered around women's emotional experience of birth and a solution to this critique: the labor support role is a complement to existing clinical roles within the current system of medicalized birth.[4]

Doula organizations and individual doulas acknowledge that some maternity care clinicians, especially labor and delivery nurses, support women some of the time. However, this

---

3 Many doulas offer a sliding scale fee. Doulas in New York City and Los Angeles areas may charge as much as $2,000 and more for their services. Often, these services include extras, such as massage, aromatherapy, hypno-birthing, childbirth education classes, or postpartum care follow-up. Some doulas do not charge a fee prior to certification.

4 Since over 99% of births occur in hospitals, we are emphasizing these births. The role of a doula at a home birth is less a critique of midwifery care as it is an acknowledgement that an unmedicated birth requires a great deal of emotional and physical support. In many home births, the midwife may rest or sleep in another room while labor continues normally.

is just one aspect of the nursing role, and nurses are increasingly required to complete routine documentation tasks, care for multiple patients, and focus on clinical situations. Nurses, midwives, and physicians, as clinical providers, are unable to continuously attend to and prioritize women's emotional and physical comfort throughout the entire course of labor and birth. Doulas, on the other hand, have defined their role to do precisely that in order to increase women's emotional satisfaction with their childbirth experiences, whatever the circumstances, wherever they occur, whether at a hospital, birth center, or home.

The vast majority of doulas embrace the midwifery model of care, which posits birth as a normal physiological event with women as active participants (Rooks, 1997). Doulas entered the world of hospital-based childbirth as ambassadors of a birth philosophy not often practiced, and frequently unseen by today's mainstream obstetric providers. Since the doula's emergence into maternity care in the early 1990s, between 3% to 6% of women have doulas at their births, and there has been an increase in the number of U.S. births attended by midwives, with the proportion of vaginal births attended by Certified Nurse Midwives, or CNMs, reaching an all-time high of 11.4% in 2009 (Declercq, 2012).

Doulas advocate evidence-based care for physiologic birth, yet are not trained to clinically recognize or treat women when their pregnancies and labors become non-normal. Thus, tensions can arise for doulas, their birthing clients, and the attending obstetric care providers when there are differing views over whether a particular procedure is medically indicated. Further, doulas, despite their allegiance to a holistic, noninterventionist philosophy of birth, are enjoined by their organizational scope of practice to respect and empower individual women's birth choices, even when these are not consistent with the doulas' beliefs or preferences. When engaged directly by pregnant women as independent practitioners, doulas are not responsible to institutional routines, yet must work within them if the birth takes place in a hospital, as 99% do. Dilemmas faced by doulas will be addressed further in this book, with the understanding that while doulas play an important role in the humanization of medicalized birth, their presence alone cannot be expected to fix the system.

The Current U.S. Maternity Care System

The current system of U.S. maternity care is often described as a perinatal paradox. Despite spending more per capita than other industrialized countries, the United States ranks 50th globally in terms of maternal mortality (Amnesty International, 2010). In addition, the U.S. ranks below many industrialized nations in infant mortality rates. Recognition of this is acknowledged in the sentinel alert, issued in January 2010 by The Joint Commission, the nation's oldest and largest standard-setting and accrediting body in health, warning that "current trends and evidence suggest that maternal mortality rates may be increasing in the U.S." (The Joint Commission, 2010). In response to the rising cesarean rate, which reached 32.9% in 2009, The Joint Commission cautions, "Despite the rising c-section rate, no population health benefits have been realized" (The Joint Commission, 2011).

Since the 1980s, doulas have joined childbirth educators, homebirth midwives, and other maternity-care advocates in asserting that much in current obstetric practice does not follow evidence-based research, and indeed, utilizes many procedures in circumstances where they are not medically necessary and may cause harm (Goer & Romano, 2012; Sakala & Corry, 2008). Within the overall context of increasing medical interventions, worsening maternal and infant-health outcomes, and higher rates of postpartum mood and anxiety disorders, doulas (as well as childbirth educators) have emerged as ambassadors of evidence-based childbirth, arguing that greater attention and commitment to the normalcy of childbirth will improve maternity outcomes for women and their babies.

Doula Stories of Birth

While birth stories are seemingly everywhere—under scrutiny by scholars and pregnant women, on the Internet, in the news, on television reality and talk shows, in books, and everyday conversations among friends and neighbors[5]—the doula's story of birth is yet untold. Birth stories bring families and strangers together in an uneasy mixture of intimacy and terror and open new avenues for their retelling. The uninvited birth story is often told to the pregnant woman and is the subject of letters to newspaper advice columnists, as well as childbirth advice books. The uninvited story, often describing a less-than-optimal experience, is dismissed as a "horror" story, or "old wives' tale," and recipients of such stories are advised to "disregard them" by advice columnists or caring friends. Cultural theorist Della Pollock describes being approached late in her first pregnancy by a woman in the produce section of the supermarket who gave a dramatic, uninvited account of her physically traumatic birth, and her response:

> This stranger's strange story became part of my body, my experience ... and, as I listened to her, I accepted the burden of this unimagined and unimaginable experience and, with it, the possibility of a new kind of pleasure, a pleasure drawing me toward a place unkempt with desire, short of social convention, constrained only by a deeper, tacit contract that stipulated she would tell, and I would listen—and bear her story to others (Pollock, 1999, p. 3).

---

5 Books featuring birth stories: (Doran & Caron, 2010, 2012; Faldet & Fitton, 1997; Gaskin, 1977/1990, 2003; Giglio, 1999; Kitzinger, 1989). Scholars analyzing birth stories: (Cosslett, 1994; Davis-Floyd, 1992/2004; Klassen, 2001; Oakley, 1979; Pollock, 1999).

Pollock's analysis of birth stories as performance highlights their shifting centers, multiple subjectivities, and their public emphasis on the comic-heroic narrative. She notes that these narratives:

> may be [complicit] with the system they otherwise often reject...directly and indirectly, they may support the norms—the desires and expectations for a "normal" birth—enforced by medical practice (Pollock, 1999, p. 6).

For the most part, Pollock says, these stories do not offer a viable alternative to medicalized birth; the majority of women portray themselves as passive recipients of medical interventions whether they credit the medical efforts as unnecessary and unwanted or as lifesaving and desired.

Women's stories of birth may be framed and told differently when doulas are present. Doulas are accepted, indeed embraced, by many expectant couples as virtual strangers at births in part because they promise a familiarity with the liminal or "in-between" experience that birth represents for most people, and because the woman becomes the center of the experience. Other than watching births via media portrayals, few people have been present throughout an entire labor and birth. For most people, birth is a black box through which a pregnant friend or daughter passes and comes out the other side a new mother. In the telling of a typical birth story, the ending is known, and the woman, or couple, has come through the experience, usually with a healthy baby, no matter what happened at the birth.[6] Doula services are overwhelmingly appreciated and praised by women after their births because the stories told by doulas highlight women's efforts while most family stories center

---

6 While most births do result in healthy babies, we acknowledge that this is mostly true among the typical clientele served by most doulas: white, privately insured, married women who are in good health and who have middle-to-high socioeconomic status.

around the baby (Koumouitzes-Douvia & Carr, 2006).

Doula care is not preparation for birth, but an interactional accomplishment of labor support by non-medically trained women during childbirth. Doulas enter medical institutions with the goals of emphasizing emotional over technological triumphs and affirming the woman's act of giving birth, rather than the physician's role in delivering the baby. Doulas articulate the need for triumph in a medicalized system overly focused on institutional routines, including numerous procedures which doulas often describe as "non-medically indicated interventions." These interventions include routine intravenous fluid lines (IVs), continuous electronic fetal monitoring (EFM), and restrictions on movement and eating during labor that doulas (and others) contend are routinely implemented in hospital birth, yet lack a strong evidence base for normal, healthy women in labor (Budin, 2007).

Birth in medicalized systems typically results in stories that emphasize risk, danger, and the primary role of the obstetrician. Doulas attempt, with varying degrees of success, to influence how women are treated within this system. The story the doula tells may also influence how women and their partners remember that birth, as well as the stories that will be told to friends, family members, and even strangers in the supermarket. The doula's story of birth is thus generating interest, curiosity, and desire as her message emerges from the cacophony of conflicting advice and heated debates over medicalized childbirth in the United States today.

Aims of this Book

Overall, this book documents the development of the doula's role as an emerging occupational niche within maternity care. It examines how the doula evolved from a cultural practice of woman-attended childbirth to a paid caregiving occupation. It describes why women become doulas, the meanings they give to their experiences, and how they negotiate the dilemmas embedded within doula practice. Sociologist Christine Morton analyzes the meanings and dilemmas of the doula role for doulas and their organizations from the stories that doulas told her during her research interviews. The personal narratives, edited by Elayne Clift, are provided as a complement to Morton's chapters that offer sociological insights on doula care. The goals of the book are to provide a social history of doulas, capture current experience and meaning of doula care, and to encourage critical reflection on the doula's place in maternity care today and in the future.

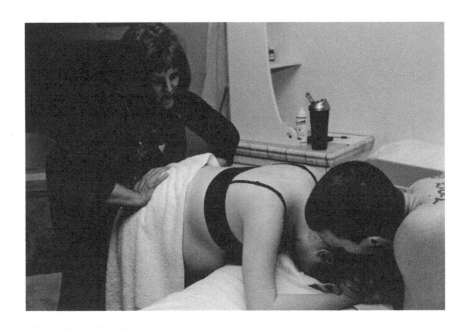

Photo 6. The doula performs a comfort measure known as the "double hip squeeze," while the woman's partner gives encouragement during a contraction.
Photo by Kyndal May.

Personal Story

THE BLESSING WAY
Liz Wilson

The greatest gift of three doula-supported births was the ability to keep the process of birth true to me. When we got pregnant, my husband and I wanted the outcomes that everyone desires: healthy baby, healthy mother, healthy family. But just as the baby that emerges is absolutely unique, so is the story of each birth. These stories describe the process that brought this new life into the world. They become charged particles, positive and negative, in the matter of family lore.

Although I almost qualified as one of "advanced maternal age" (mid-30s) for my first pregnancy, I had not heard many birth stories that conveyed strength and empowerment from a woman's perspective. My own mother's seven stories were told as if all that mattered was the baby, not that she was abandoned in a cellar room of the hospital during labor, over-drugged and unable to push, and then left alone again after the birth of my oldest brother (1950); or that she asked to feel nothing for my birth, her seventh delivery (1963), and then almost died from the anesthesia. Just because the baby was healthy, clearly, did not make the process of no consequence. Her stories became cautionary tales for me. It was not until I had experienced the emotional cacophony of new motherhood myself that I wondered if in her retelling, she muted the emotional impact of these harrowing experiences.

I was fortunate to have a group of women, other new moms, whom I connected with soon after the birth of my first child. We shared our stories, our all-over-the-map emotions, the challenges of our physical reconstruction, and we helped each other through the constant redefinition of our lives as mothers. Every Thursday morning for almost five years, we entered our "Red Tent." Now when my children clamor to hear their birth stories, I have become aware that choosing a doula allowed me to be a more powerful author of these stories, and a positive contributor to the ethos that shapes and forms the lives of my children.

I admit that I was not consciously thinking about story making when pregnant and learning about birth. All I knew was that I wanted to have some say in the process. But this was the tricky part. I imagined myself sitting at a table with the formidable forces of Mother Nature and Modern Medicine, and then with my husband, an obstetrician/gynecologist. He did this for a living. I feared all these forces would subsume me during birth unless I found some support for my own process. Mother Nature was going to start, and not stop, until there was a baby; Modern Medicine was going to follow hospital protocol and do its usual interventions unless guided otherwise; and my husband would be, well, at work in a zone totally familiar to him, but not to me. How was I going to hold my own? I was going to be surrounded by my husband's co-workers—some of whom I would meet for the first time half naked, groaning, and in pain. I knew I needed some reinforcement. Enter Paige, our doula.

Paige helped to constructively and peaceably partner Mother Nature, Modern Medicine, my husband John, and myself during three birth experiences that were richly and comfortably our own, and which continue to bless and empower me and my family.

I became pregnant for the first time during John's second year of OB/GYN residency at University Hospitals in Cleveland, Ohio in 1996. Although I had regularly heard about all sorts of births for over two years from the physician's perspective, I had no preconceived (literally) notion of how I wanted to give birth. It was not until I began to show in my second trimester that the inevitability of this life in me making its way out sent me voraciously in search of information about the birth process. I read books and grilled my husband on the current standard of care. I soon realized that my quiet bent toward medical non-intervention, such as not taking cold medicine because it might mask what my body is trying to "say" to me, was leading me down the "hear me roar" path of natural childbirth.

As a coach of many years and a life-long athlete, I could not help but look at childbirth as a physical and mental challenge, much like a competition or a race. On the "big" day, it had a distinct starting point, a process in which time was a factor, and an outcome known only in its generalities, not in the details. I was sure that choosing natural childbirth would be one of the biggest mind/body challenges I would ever face. I imagined the culmination of a race—the pain of exhaustion, feeling ready to puke, falling down and giving up. I knew I had to be really prepared, but I also needed a great support team. It took one type of teamwork to get pregnant, but it was going to take a wholly different kind to bring the baby home.

I began making phone calls to different birthing class programs. Paige, who also taught the Bradley Natural Childbirth education classes, was the first person I finally felt could speak to the experience of giving birth in a way that resonated with my hopes and values. Paige spoke about how important it is to know the details of the physical process, the emotional markers of labor, and the teamwork with the husband, nurses, and doctor. I got this. I likened it to being in season preparing for games: get in shape, do your exercises, eat well, stay in tune with your body, know your teammates, know what you're up against, and what variables you might face. Get straight on what you can and cannot control. John would say OBs commonly gave the eye roll when their patients would write out detailed, proscriptive birth plans because often these were the women who ended up with the most intervention. I tested him on the necessity and impact of medical intervention in the birth process; he was comfortable with it as long as it had the latest evidence-based scientific acceptance. For me, working with what nature designed seemed the optimal choice for my children, myself, and then, in the bigger picture, for my family. John knew natural childbirth had to be my decision. He had a lot of faith in me. But he was comfortable with medical intervention; he took cold medicine.

Paige, it turned out, was a doula as well as a childbirth educator. It did not take much explanation of the role of a doula for me to know that this was what I wanted—the knowledge, wisdom, and training of this very cool childbirth educator with us in the delivery room. For all three of my births, Paige was my advocate and helped me feel strong in my position to have natural childbirth amidst institutions where this was not the norm and the majority of deliveries were anesthetized. She took care of me and tended to my needs throughout labor and delivery with knowing massage, coaching, cooling washcloths, humor, position changes, and exchanges with John, the nurses, and doctors. Her constant presence allowed me to keep my energy focused inside on relaxation, breathing, and helping the baby out. She worked seamlessly alongside John, letting him be with me in the ways that were true to him. His expertise, calm, and confidence were of enormous comfort to me; if anything went awry, I trusted him implicitly to do what was needed for me and the baby. I did not, however, trust that he would know the best counter-pressure spot to relieve my intense contractions. John was my rock; Paige was my warm blanket.

At first, I felt like such a rebel choosing a doula-supported birth. For many, the notion that I would want or need anyone besides my husband as support for me during birth was a novel concept; but if we examine a bigger slice of time, having husbands attend birth is much more novel than having a woman support another woman in labor. A doula is a known and a constant, a steady presence for the mother during labor and delivery. Nowadays, in the other cast of characters, nurses may change shifts, doctors check in and out; even spouses, the close friend, or family member can experience fatigue in the marathon of labor, and the emotional exertion—both in supporting their spouses and maintaining their own equilibrium in this heated, primal event. Paige helped me keep myself in a kind of balance: a participant in the nature of birth while amidst the back-up of modern medical technology. Birth, like death, is a dramatic affirmation that we are indeed nature—we are subject to its cycles, to its woes and wonders. Birth reveals both women's power and vulnerability in nature. It is a time to take great stock and great care. I am grateful that each birth was an intimate experience that connected me soulfully with my husband, doula, doctor, and nurses, but also with myself and nature.

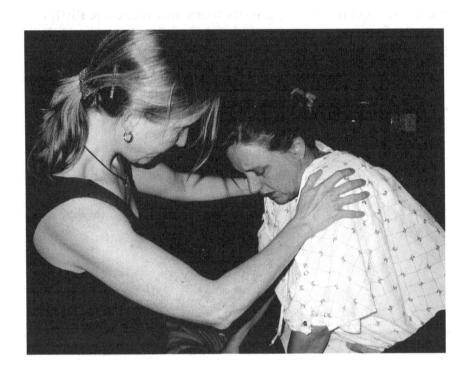

Photo 7. The doula offers encouragement to the laboring woman during a contraction.
Photo by Kyndal May.

Chapter One

The Birth of Doulas: A Social History[1]

Women and men have always found it hard to comprehend and to convey to each other what they feel experiencing childbirth, and what they see witnessing it.

Margarete Sandelowski[2]

In spite of, or perhaps because of the difficulty in conveying the power and mysteries of childbirth, there has been an explosion of scholarly and popular writing on the topic in the past 40 years, the latter fueled in large measure by the Internet. Less examined is how woman-to-woman support during childbirth transformed from a kin and community-centered relationship to a mainly fee-for-service transaction among relative strangers.

Doula care emerged as a unique response to the changing social and medical contexts of childbirth support in the United States in the late 1980s through early 1990s. Childbirth support is defined here as the use of interventive technologies (medical, herbal, technological), the social provision of physical assistance, and the culturally shared meanings at-

---

1 This chapter is based on the author's sociological research on the history and experiences of doulas in the United States. The methodology is described in the Appendix.

2 Sandelowski, M. (1984). *Pain, pleasure and American childbirth: From the twilight sleep to the Read method, 1914-1960.* Westport, CT: Greenwood Press, p. xiii.

tached to childbirth and mothering. Throughout history and across cultures, human societies have had childbirth support systems that addressed the issues of facing the unknown—encountering fear, pain, and possibly death, as they awaited the existence of a new social member. These three dimensions of childbirth support have gradually been altered since the 1930s, when they were densely concentrated within women's social networks. Since the 1960s, however, they have become widely distributed among a variety of social actors, technologies, and locations. In particular, labor support—the provision of emotional, physical, and informational support—became a specifically delimited role in the form of the doula.

The contingencies of time, physiology, and culture are interwoven into the history of childbirth support. Pregnancy, and labor in particular, are liminal, or "in-between" states that are temporally bound. Women don't remain pregnant forever; labor ultimately ends in some way. Death for either the woman or the infant is a potential, if currently rare, outcome, at least in industrialized countries; but continuing to be pregnant, or continuing to be in labor indefinitely are not options. The myriad histories and accounts of the changing structural arrangements surrounding childbirth support reveal a variety of ideological and cultural meanings about birth practices, materials, and meanings within societies and among scholars. This is inevitable, as anthropologist Brigitte Jordan, so eloquently writes:

> In some senses the physiology of birth is universally the same—yet parturition is accomplished in strikingly different ways by different groups of people. We know from cross-cultural evidence that birth is everywhere treated as a marked life-crisis event. As such, this period is everywhere a candidate for consensual shaping and social patterning. In most societies, birth, and the immediate postpartum period, are considered a time of vulnerability for mother and child; indeed, frequently

a time of ritual danger for the entire family or community. In order to deal with this danger, and the existential uncertainty associated with birth, people tend to produce a set of internally consistent and mutually dependent practices and beliefs, which are designed to manage the physiologically and socially problematic aspects of parturition in a way that makes sense in that particular cultural context. It is not surprising, therefore, that—whatever the details of a particular birthing system—its practitioners will tend to see it as the best way, the right way, indeed the way to bring a child into the world. For these reasons we find that within any given system, birth practices appear packaged into a relatively uniform, systematic, standardized, ritualized, even morally required routine. We acknowledge such recognizable, culturally specific configurations of practices and beliefs when we talk, for example, about "Western obstetrics," or the various "ethno-obstetrics" of traditional societies (Jordan, 1983/1993, p. 2).

Jordan was writing in the early 1980s, just as major challenges to American obstetric practice were beginning to emerge, and she was interested in comparing birthing cultures, even variations within "Western" obstetrics, by looking at birth in the United States, Holland, Sweden, and the Yucatán. Compared to the latter three cultures, the history of childbirth support in the United States changed dramatically within a relatively short period of time. Historians, evolutionary anthropologists, and social scientists have examined multiple factors, and sometimes conflicting explanations, for the dramatic changes in childbirth support seen in the United States. According to Barbara Katz Rothman, the history of maternity care is the history of midwifery, and the history of obstetric care is the fall of midwifery (Donegan, 1978; Donnison, 1977; Rooks, 1997; Rothman, 1982/1991; Sullivan & Weitz, 1988). This view highlights changes in birth attendants while other analyses focus on women's experience and the presence of fathers in the birth room (Leavitt, 1986, 2009), the changing ideology of birth (Kahn, 1995; Sandelowski, 1984; Simonds, Rothman, & Norman, 2006), or on the medicalization process (Cassidy, 2006; Caton, 1999; Perkins, 2003; Shorter, 1991; Witz, 1992; Wolf, 2009).

The medicalization of childbirth has been critiqued for contributing to the fall of midwifery care (Donegan, 1978; Donnison, 1977; Leavitt, 1986; Rothman, 1982/1991; Simonds, Rothman & Norman, 2006; Sullivan & Weitz, 1988; Wertz & Wertz, 1977) as well as supplanting alternative discourses, such as midwifery, or women-centered healthcare (Arney, 1982; Treichler, 1990). Perhaps the most trenchant critique has been the manner in which obstetrics operates to minimize or deny birthing women's agency in the service of the technocratic view of birth managed by maternity care clinicians, primarily obstetricians (Davis-Floyd, 1992/2004; Murphy-Lawless, 1999; Rothman, 1982/1991). Among more radical thinkers, this impulse has been attributed to patriarchal desire to control the means of reproduction and/or commodify its various components (Kahn, 1995; O'Brien, 1981; Rich, 1995; Rothman, 1982/1991).[3] The ongoing challenges and contests over professional authority, changes in and access to technology, and the right to provide and define the content of childbirth support to pregnant women has a complex, contentious history in the U.S.

The existing literature, while familiar to many, can be examined through the lens of labor support to see how this role became crystallized in the form of the "doula." Although variation in particular childbirth practices existed in the "traditional" period (up to 1930 or so), it was primarily women in community networks who routinely provided childbirth support in all its facets (Leavitt, 1986; Wertz & Wertz, 1977).

---

3 This radical displacement of midwifery care did not occur in European countries, such as Great Britain, Denmark, or the Netherlands, for example (Sullivan & Weitz, 1988).

However, as social childbirth practices changed between 1930 and 1960, the fragmentation of childbirth support began with biomedical experts claiming authority over pregnant women's health and childbirth outcomes and moving birth to the hospital. The next decades are characterized by the emergence of various political, professional and consumer negotiations around childbirth practices, which called for women to be "awake and aware" and take an active role in their birth experiences. In the past 40 years, there has been increasing accommodation to medicalized childbirth support as well as renewed interest in merging holistic and medical approaches (Davis-Floyd, 2001). It is in this period we see the emergence of the doula as a particular, specialized role in providing non-medical (emotional, physical, and informational) support to birthing women.

Traditional Childbirth Support:
Women's Networks of Care

Like all birth stories, the birth story of the doula is context-specific, with different versions depending on the teller and the listener (Cosslett, 1994). When doulas make the connection between their current practice and historical precedent, they note the anthropological evidence suggesting the sociality of childbirth results from the physical challenges presented by human upright postures and large brains in newborn infants (Hrdy, 1999; Trevathan, 1987). Doula trainers often introduce written and visual examples from archeological evidence of stone carvings and statues of birthing women surrounded by other women. They cite anthropological data indicating that in all but one of 128 cultures studied, a family member or friend remains with a woman throughout labor and birth (Trevathan, 1987). Doulas and their organizations claim to continue this tradition of woman-supported birth, recreating it from historical, cultural, and women's ongoing everyday practices. This tradition, they claim, has been interrupted due to an anomalous period in American childbirth history where medicalized, hospitalized birthing women have been bereft of supportive care by lay women knowledgeable about and sensitive to women's emotional experiences of childbirth.

Doulas turn to history, and to women's subjective experience of medicalized birth, to argue for the universality of women's emotional needs in labor. Many doulas draw on selected elements from the traditional period of childbirth support to claim a collective kinship with these women-centered networks (Blue, 1994; Simkin, 1992b). The turn of the 20th century was a time when most American women gave birth at home, attended by their close female relatives and friends who brought with them generations' worth of everyday knowledge and experience (Bogdan, 1978; Leavitt, 1986). Childbirth was a social event and historians have well documented that childbirth support "included women who were not members of the family and who were not paid to attend. Many of them acted on the basis of reciprocity, in the expectation that others would care for them in their turn" (Wertz & Wertz, 1977, p. 4).

The shift from midwife-attended homebirth to physician-attended hospital birth occurred fairly rapidly.

As late as 1900, half of all the children born in a given year in the United States were delivered with the help of a midwife attendant. Yet, by 1930 midwife-attended births had dropped to less than 15 percent of all births in the United States, and most of these were in the South (Borst, 1995, p.1).

Not only had midwife-attended births declined, home-based support networks, in the form of community women, were also in decline. These changes were facilitated as physicians sought a role within pregnancy and childbirth, first by attending women in their homes, and then in hospitals. The rapid shift in birth location in the 1940s and 1950s dramatically altered the pre-eminent role of women's social networks. As long as the birth remained in the home:

> Women could afford to ask medical experts to take care of some of the technical aspects of childbirth precisely because they had their support group in place to take care of the crucial emotional bonds associated with sharing the experience of giving birth to the next generation. The support network that women gathered around them at the time of their confinements provided the necessary base for women's ability to resist some medical practices and to keep considerable control in their own hands (Leavitt, 1986, p. 210).

Birth historians show how female relatives often came from great distances to attend to their sister, cousin, or daughter during her lying-in period (Leavitt, 1986; Lewis, 1986; Rothman, 1982/1991; Scholten, 1985). The social provision of physical support included an intimate understanding of how to provide hands-on physical care, as well as how to manage the everyday needs of the household during the woman's lying-in period (Wertz & Wertz, 1977). This encompassed a variety of tasks, with physical and emotional consequences for the birthing woman: cooking, cleaning, laundry, tending the heat source, reassuring and caring for the woman's husband and other children. This support was many-to-one, with a focus on the individual as she lived in her own home, among her intimate relationships. Many of these community women were also familiar with the use of the herbal remedies or physical techniques of midwives. Thus, the experiential wisdom collectively held by the women in attendance could often address and resolve problematic birth situations. The interwoven nature of women-controlled technologies and support were seen as significant for the health and well-being of the laboring woman

> The potential medical value of the psychological support these female friends offered should not be undervalued; the presence of women provided particular reassurance during a woman's first birth, helping her to relax and thus to ease her pain (Wertz & Wertz, 1977, p. 5).

However, once the location of birth shifted, this support network was ruptured. In some ways, this shift addressed very real fears and risks associated with childbirth at that time, but in doing so, it replaced the community values of supportive social networks with the scientific values of authority and technology, including medications for pain relief.

At the same time, women's social networks were disintegrating with the rapid urbanization characterizing the early 20th century, thus contributing to the social fragmentation of women-centered childbirth support (Leavitt, 1986). By the end of this traditional period, the practice of lay woman-to-woman support, via midwifery and informal social networks, had been replaced by professionalized medical and nursing care in hospitals.

Modern Childbirth Support—Professionalized Medical Care (1930s-1960s)

As the shift to hospital births became more widespread across the country, the traditional form of childbirth support was radically changed. Now the technologies, physical support, and meanings given to birth were incorporated into increasingly medicalized and professionalized arrangements.

Physicians, holding the promise of safety and sterility, moved to adopt practices and technologies that quickly became rigid and lacking in compassion for women's subjective experiences of birth. Hospitals moved from providing medical and moral services to urban poor women to actively courting patients in their desire to attract wealthy and middle-class clientele (Leavitt, 1986; Starr, 1982).

Many first-person accounts of women's experiences document the fear and pain associated with childbirth in the first half of the 20th century (Leavitt, 1986; Lewis, 1986). Physicians and hospitals offered promises of relief from pain and potential infection in part to address women's fears. The growing use of, and demand for, "Twilight Sleep," an amnesiac mixture of scopolamine and morphine, which left women with no memories of giving birth, may be seen as one response. As Leavitt notes:

Most women did not view the stay in the hospital as a time when they lost important parts of the traditional birth experience, but rather as a time when they gained protection for life and health, aspects of birth that had been elusive and uncertain in the past (Leavitt, 1986, p. 181).

However, women were divided between those who actively formed the Twilight Sleep Association, seeking complete pain relief (and no memory of the event), and those who wanted to be conscious and use as little pain medication as possible. One female physician caused an uproar at the 1936 American Medical Association symposium on obstetrics when she stated:

In my opinion, no woman whether intelligent or unintelligent, modern or old-fashioned, wants the birth of a baby a blank in her memory. Certainly, none will wish to be relieved of pain at the risk of harm to the baby (Edwards & Waldorf, 1984, p.1).

Dr. Gertrude Nielsen believed the high maternal death rate at the time was in part due to the growing use of analgesics and she drew upon her own experience of giving birth to three children without drugs to argue her case for a more natural, less fear-based view. The ensuing debate in *The New York Times* highlighted many issues still relevant and controversial today, some 75 years later: the safety of anesthetic drugs for both the woman and the baby; the link between fear, knowledge, and pain in labor; women's right to full information about risks of choosing medication for pain relief; their ability to make those decisions; and structural support for whatever decision they make.

As in every age and culture, the social organization of childbirth support is influenced by prevailing views on women's social roles. During the 1930s and 1940s, Freud's writings sparked an interest in psychosomatic medicine among physicians. The meaning of childbirth support in this period incorporated a Freudian perspective on women's emotions. Emotions and feelings were seen as important, although in this framework, they were pathologized and the root of any problem was believed to lie in the individual. Addressing these emotions was seen as a way to pre-empt hysteria, depression, and Oedipal conflicts. As more women gave birth in the hospital, the obstetric nurse was viewed as one way to meet women's emotional needs in childbirth.

Nursing emerged as a separate occupation in the late 19th century through the 1950s, as the "physician's lieutenant" (Sandelowski, 1984). The modern role of the doula is strikingly similar to Sandelowski's description of the obstetric nurse during the advent of psychosomatic medicine in the 1930s— one of the few historical examinations of this occupational role. Little research has been done on the historical or current role of the obstetric nurse, but in Sandelowski's history, the obstetric nurse:

... primarily protected the childbearing woman from the hazards of misinformation, anxiety, and loneliness ... it was primarily the nurse who comforted, counseled, and cared for the childbearing woman, providing her with the most constant professional attention of any caregiver in the maternity cycle (Sandelowski, 1984, p. 61).

Obstetric nurses emerged as a distinctly American version of their European counterpart—trained midwives—without this title and without challenging physician's leadership role. The nurse's role was to support and augment, but not replace the physician, in responsibility or authority. Physicians courted nurses and absolutely depended on them to attend to patients, but were clearly afraid of nurses' potential for dislodging them from their preeminent place in maternity care both by virtue of the experiential authority and their emotional connection to women. Yet Sandelowski argues that "physicians really had nothing to fear from nurses who accepted the demanding, but obsequious role that physicians and prevailing cultural norms concerning the proper role of women in healthcare expected them to play" (Sandelowski, 1984, p. 65).[4]

Nurses then, as today, support and care for laboring women both emotionally and medically, managing the administration of medications, monitoring the health of the woman and her baby, and knowing when to call the physician. Notwithstanding the marked reduction in maternal mortality between 1937 and 1945, by many accounts hospital-based maternity care became increasingly regimented, so that by the late 1940s, "nurses began to appear less like sisterly companions in labor and more like unfeeling robots" (Sandelowski, 1984, p. 68).

Birthing women were now surrounded by and subject to the authority of professional medical and nursing staff in hospitals with new "scientific" ideas about birth and child-

---

4 Many would argue that the same is true for doulas today, explaining why they have been welcomed by some physicians and hospitals.

care rather than among a community of like-minded women. Nursing care gradually shifted from a model of one-on-one to one-on-many over this period. Hospitals largely replaced home as the site of most births, but also kept women in their midst for the first two weeks after birth, distancing them from their social support networks and their husbands, and establishing institutional authority over proper infant care, especially with regard to timed feedings of artificial baby milks.

The medicalization of motherhood in this way also worked to assimilate large numbers of immigrant mothers into "modern" American mothering and childrearing practices (Cowan & Cowan, 1996; Litt, 2000). The messages surrounding the meaning of birth were extended to mothering and largely focused on values associated with "progress" and "modernity": cleanliness, sterility, and scientific expertise over all matters relating to social reproduction. At the same time, the moral meaning of pain shifted from an emphasis on religious messages about bearing humanity's sin through childbirth to pain as something one could, and should, avoid. Into this milieu came the first rumblings of discontent, with natural childbirth philosophies and methods imported from England and France.[5]

British physician Grantly Dick-Read had been practicing obstetrics for more than ten years when he wrote *Natural Childbirth* in 1930, published in 1933. Dick-Read's philosophy and experiences became the rallying cry of a movement in the United States, when it was published as *Childbirth without Fear: The Principles and Practices of Natural Childbirth* in 1944. However, the introduction of Dick-Read's ideas within the American context of institutionalized hospital birth meant that women who tried to experience "childbirth without fear" were still left unsupported, alone, and in the midst of insti-

---

5 "Natural childbirth" has a vague and uncertain meaning, depending on who is using it. The term was easily redefined and co-opted by physicians to mean vaginal births (even with pain medications and/or instrument deliveries) as well as unmedicated birth with no interventions (including the IV drip). The term natural childbirth is used here to refer to unmedicated, low-intervention, vaginal births.

tutional procedures designed for the ease of the physician. It was easier, according to sociologist Barbara Katz Rothman, for society to view women who attempted to use Dick-Read's method as individual failures, rather than acknowledging their concerns as valid and rethinking institutional arrangements of childbirth (Rothman, 1982/1991).

The modern period of social childbirth practices changed how various components of childbirth support had been structured, leaving patients dissatisfied with the technological incursion into the social provision of physical support. Women eagerly sought some interventive technologies; these initially seemed to address their fears and compensate for the loss of social support networks, but there were real costs. The dehumanizing practices embedded in the wide scale application of such technologies (including women being physically strapped to tables, subjected to routine enemas and pubic shaves, and long periods of separation from their newborns) had physically and emotionally traumatic effects on women and their families.

This was vividly illustrated in the outpouring of letters published in the *Ladies' Home Journal* in 1958 in response to a complaint by an anonymous registered nurse detailing the cruelty and abuses she had witnessed in maternity wards. The *Journal* editors invited reader responses, which verified the original complaints and cited additional problems. Letters written by childbearing women, nurses, and physicians attested to the reality of women being strapped to delivery tables and left for hours; births delayed to await the physician's arrival; and callous treatment and verbal abuse by nurses and doctors alike. Physicians and nurses consulted by the *Journal* did not deny these charges, but argued that hospital administrators could and should be the ones responsible for change. In December 1958, the *Journal* published a list of recommendations to improve hospital childbirth conditions, including the right for husbands to accompany their wives in labor.

In the midst of this discussion and debate, childbirth reform activists began to organize and teach natural childbirth methods. One such group began in Seattle—the Association for Childbirth Education (ACE)—and although they advocated breastfeeding, rooming in, and husbands at births, "they took care to explain that they weren't attacking medical management of birth, nor the doctors' right to control, but only urging modifications" (Edwards & Waldorf, 1984, p. 61).

Nursing historian Margarete Sandelowski describes the dominant approach taken by most natural childbirth advocates at the time.

> Natural Childbirth (NC), in the 1940s and 1950s, was distinctively non-feminist, if not anti-feminist, and pro-medical in control of the childbirth arena. It is simply inaccurate to politicize the early NC movement by depicting women and physicians as adversaries on two sides of the NC argument. The trend toward psychosomatic medicine, and women's increasing demand to be satisfied, converged in the NC movement ... Childbearing women simply wanted to be satisfied in childbirth and to be treated more humanely by their caregivers, and it was certainly in physicians' interest to help them achieve this (Sandelowski, 1984, p. 136).

Most observers agree that reform efforts focused on educating women about the process of childbirth, granting fathers the permission to be present at births, and helping women through childbirth. None of these reforms challenged the ultimate authority of the physician. Rather, as sociologist Barbara Katz Rothman notes that "prepared childbirth tried to humanize medical management—not to do away with the medical approach, but to make it more pleasant for women, more responsive to their needs" (Rothman 1982/1991, p.170).

As we see next, maternity care advocates continued their reform efforts around humanizing births in the medical settings, while at the same time a burgeoning midwifery movement would emerge to provide an out-of-hospital alternative.

Reformed Childbirth Support—Safety and Satisfaction in Birth (1960s-1980s)

Ever since birth moved out of women's homes and into the hospital, birthing women, individually and collectively, have been trying to recapture some of what they lost, at the same time maintaining what they have won.

Judith Walzer Leavitt[6]

During the "reformed" period, various political, professional, and consumer-advocacy groups emerged to contest the more medicalized aspects of childbirth support. Their critiques focused on women's experiences of being restrained and rendered unconscious. The alternative was for women to be "awake and aware" and to take an active role in the birth. Concerns were raised about the physical and psychological impacts of medicalized childbirth on infants, as well. Research on mother-infant bonding provided scientific legitimacy to some consumer demands, such as rooming-in with the newborn. Technological changes in childbirth support occurred simultaneously, with the phasing out of Twilight Sleep, and its replacement with a spinal anesthetic that allowed the woman to remain conscious throughout the labor, although not necessarily during the birth itself. These new medical technologies, however, resulted in increased monitoring and the routine use of other interventions, such as forceps.

6 Leavitt, J. W. (1986). *Brought to bed: Childbearing in America, 1750-1950*. Oxford, UK: Oxford University Press, p. 214.

During the 1950s and 1960s, medical authority was not greatly challenged by consumer demands for childbirth reform. Even while providing alternative breastfeeding information and advice to that available from physicians, the founders of La Leche League recognized the continued value of alliance with biomedical authority. From the organization's beginning in 1956, its advisory boards always included physicians (Ward, 2000). However, this time period also saw a resurgence of licensed and nurse midwifery, in particular, among activists who were not satisfied with leaving birth in the hands of physicians. Childbirth education, begun with the goals to educate and empower women, became quickly incorporated into hospital practice, losing its independence and potential for a more radical critique of medicalized childbirth (Declercq, 1983; Edwards & Waldorf, 1984; Rothman, 1982/1991; Sandelowski, 1984).

Gradually, it became clear to childbirth reformers that hospitals and doctors were not going to alter their practices around the assumption of "normal" birth. Despite some gains—fathers could be present during labor, if not birth; rooming-in with the baby; reduced drug dosages; and independent childbirth classes—the reform efforts were up against powerful forces (Edwards & Waldorf, 1984). New pharmaceuticals, technological changes (fueled by military-industrial resources), and profits derived from the routine use of costly machinery consolidated the relationship between the health industry, insurance companies, and the government during this period (Perkins, 2003). In the provision of "reformed" childbirth support, then, technocratic imperatives were dominant (Davis-Floyd, 1992/2004). Medicalized childbirth became firmly entrenched as the norm although still critiqued for its failure to provide adequate social and emotional support.

Ferdinand Lamaze was a French physician who had been influenced by the idea of psychoprophylaxis, i.e., conditioning the mind to influence the bodily experience of pain. After observing Russian obstetric wards using this method,

Lamaze developed it further and published his results in *Painless Childbirth* in 1956. Marjorie Karmel is credited with introducing this method in 1959 to the United States in her book, *Thank you Dr. Lamaze: A Mother's Experience with Painless Childbirth*, which detailed her own experiences in Paris. The French model was centered on a *monitrice*: a licensed or registered nurse trained in the Lamaze method of natural childbirth. The *monitrice* worked extensively with women prenatally, training them in the method, and attended their births. However, the introduction of the Lamaze method in the United States did not emphasize this role. Although some nurses who taught Lamaze classes in hospitals adopted this role, the *monitrice* was sidelined by the emphasis on the husband as the labor coach in American Lamaze classes.

The methods and theories of Dick-Read, and later, Lamaze, gave credence to the view that women's emotional needs in labor were related to childbirth outcomes. Childbirth educators drew on this relationship and made it the cornerstone of their curriculum.

> Read called attention to the socio-emotional context in which birth takes place: he did not speak only of its psychological meaning for the individual woman. Read taught women relaxation techniques ... He stated, "No greater curse can fall upon a young woman whose first labor has commenced than the crime of enforced loneliness." Furthermore, he emphasized that women needed continual comfort and emotional support throughout labor (Rothman, 1982/1991, p. 87).

The early successes that women found following these techniques may have been the personalized attention and emotional support that was an essential component of the method (Richards, 1992; Rothman, 1982/1991). In teaching and supporting women in the use of these methods, childbirth educators found support for their growing sense that women's emotional response to their birth was critical to their subsequent perception of the birth and for the quality of their transition to mothering.

The Emotional Experience of Childbirth

Emotions are experienced and produced within specific gendered, cultural, and economic contexts (Hunter & Deery, 2008). The increasing centrality of emotions in childbirth reflects some of the paradigm shifts that were underway in psychology and counseling in the 1970s and 1980s. The following quote from Sheila Kitzinger, a prominent British social anthropologist of childbirth, reflected the sense of many at the time.

> What, in fact, do we really want? I know what I want to do. I want to help each woman to be able to trust her body, and willingly, gladly with her eyes shining, to give birth. To do this she needs not only technical know-how— though an adequate activity of response to the signal of uterine contractions is important—not only intellectual information, but a psychosexual harmony through which she can joyfully surrender her body to the creative experience. This has significance in the moments of birth, for the couple in their marriage, and for relationships within the family and society (Kitzinger, 1977, p. 53).

Childbirth educators and midwifery advocates increasingly emphasized that how women feel during childbirth is critical to their experience of that birth and to their subsequent transition to motherhood. Exactly how to accomplish the goal of women giving birth with trust and glad shining eyes was being defined in the writings and teaching of childbirth educators throughout the 1970s and 1980s.

The childbirth movement was personally empowering for many women working within it, especially within the context of the larger women's movement in the late 1970s. Within childbirth activist circles, many women who had babies in the late 1970s and early 1980s used the Lamaze method as a way to achieve their goal of unmedicated childbirth, and saw it as one route among many to empowering women. According to Henci Goer, an early birth activist, "Lamaze was an empowering movement and it has grown and changed. Much of the early childbirth education did start as part of the women's movement, but it has now been co-opted by hospitals" (H. Goer, personal communication, January 3, 2002).

However, childbirth education's potential for empowering women was barely realized before this co-optation, or not at all, according to some feminist analysts.

> It is widely held that the childbirth practices developed in the 1920s, including heavy medication, make up "traditional" childbirth, and childbirth preparation is a revolution against that tradition. That is not what happened. The childbirth preparation movement, far from being a revolution, is at most a reformation movement, working within the medical model (Rothman, 1982/1991, p. 79).

The institutionalization of childbirth education, from independent, community-based gatherings in teachers' homes to hospital-run classes led by nurses, is an important part of the doula history that has yet to be fully told. While critics of prepared childbirth have analyzed texts, especially those of Dick-Read, Lamaze, and Karmel, there are, unfortunately, few firsthand accounts from women who began teaching community childbirth education classes from the 1950s onward. This is a slice of women's history that deserves further exploration, as even histories of the women's health movement have ignored the history of childbirth advocacy (Morgen, 2002).

The increasing professionalization of childbirth education resulted in fewer independent childbirth educators offering classes. Both nurse and non-nurse educators were employed by hospitals that could provide a steady stream of students and offer a range of classes geared toward siblings and grandparents over the entire course of the pregnancy. The rise of hospital-based childbirth education was criticized by some for emphasizing accommodation to and information about hospital routines rather than providing independent information and tools for self-advocacy and empowerment in birth. Sociologist Barbara Katz Rothman noted that "natural childbirth" was quickly turned into "prepared childbirth" to meet needs of hospitalized women without challenging the doctor or hospital rules.

> Rather than being alerted to which hospital procedures are arbitrary or might be unnecessary in her case, the woman is taught instead how to ignore—"breathe through"—enemas, perineal shaves, repeated examinations, transfer from bed to stretcher, and so on. The focusing technique is thus one for dealing with the hospital, and may not be directly related to the birth experience (Rothman, 1982/1991, p. 172).

Prepared childbirth often meant preparing women for anesthesia, especially in the second stage of labor, during the birth of the baby. In essence, Barbara Katz Rothman saw Lamaze during that time as "making the woman a good—non-complaining, obedient, cooperative—patient" (Rothman, 1982/1991, p. 93). The early co-optation of childbirth education and the lack of sustained challenge to physician and biomedical authority, therefore, is partly why midwifery, or even the *monitrice*, was never taken seriously as a solution to what was wrong with American childbirth support in this "modern" period.

Labor support as a stand-alone service developed as childbirth educators began attending births of their students who were committed to natural childbirth but who had no other support person available. Other dimensions of childbirth support were still firmly entrenched within medicalized birth. Physicians were in charge of medical and technological interventions. The ease of monitoring several women simultaneously allowed nurses to be responsible for more than one patient at a time. Those women who wanted to try "natural childbirth" brought a support person with them, usually the father of the baby. Writings from this time indicate that many women were successful in achieving natural childbirth, but were still considered to be on the "fringe" of normal. Never a broad-based movement, the fragmentation, ideological differences, and organizational dynamics within childbirth reform and education certainly limited attempts to expand the membership base.[7]

Although the women's health movement grew dramatically from the mid-1970s, the influence of feminism on activists in the childbirth education movement is less clear. Just as women's health activists challenged the cultural dictate to be passive consumers of health and medical information, so too did many individual childbirth educators. The 1972 publication of *Our Bodies, Ourselves* contained women's stories, in their own words, about their health and medical experiences, and provided alternative sources of authoritative information about women's health concerns, especially childbirth. The influential *Spiritual Midwifery*, published in 1977, was less explicitly a feminist text, but no less authoritative in presenting an alternative to obstetric hegemony.

Childbirth education, midwifery, and the women's health movement contributed to the slow but steady growth of licensed (direct-entry) midwifery and certified nurse-midwifery from the 1980s onward (Rooks, 1997). This period also inspired several feminist research projects on the history of midwifery, its past struggles to achieve professional autonomy in the realm of normal childbirth, and its future promise

---

7 This also explains why there are so many organizations currently training and certifying doulas. The future of doula training and doula practice may follow this pattern of childbirth education.

for transforming current childbirth practices (Donegan, 1978; Donnison, 1977; Rooks, 1997; Rothman, 1982/1991; Sullivan & Weitz, 1988). These texts served as critical sources of information and justification for modern doulas' roles at births (Blue, 1994; Simkin, 1992b). Whether and how the childbirth reform movement actors engaged critically, or disagreed with, some of the fundamental tenets of feminist thought remains an empirical question, deserving systematic exploration.

A central concern of many in the childbirth reform movement was the impact of dehumanizing birth practices on women's emotional experiences, but also on the newborns' experience (Odent, 1984). An important development in the history of the doula role occurred when two physician researchers stumbled across the surprising (to them) finding that emotional support for laboring women improved birth outcomes, as well as increasing mother-infant bonding after premature births, their primary interest.

In 1972, pediatricians Marshall Klaus and John Kennell published a study in *The New England Journal of Medicine* showing that mothers who spent extra time with their newborns right after birth demonstrated better mothering skills, and their infants did better on development tests, than mothers and infants without such extended contact (Klaus, Jerauld, Kreger, McAlpine, Steffa, & Kennell, 1972). The "discovery" of this critical first hour after birth provided women with scientific validation for their emotional responses to hospital practices of routine mother-infant separation. The findings also provided rationale to consumer groups and hospitals to change birthing practices to allow fathers in the birthing room and to allow infants to remain with their mothers during their hospital stay rather than be taken to the central nursery.

Klaus and Kennell's findings were strongly critiqued from many angles, feminist and non-feminist alike, for methodological inadequacies, vague concept definition, lack of true control and experimental groups, and for the value judgments implied in the mother's social role (Arney, 1980; Eyer,

1992). However, the pediatricians' dramatic research findings and elaboration of bonding theory coincided with increasingly vocal childbirth activist demands for change. Among other things, bonding theory provided a framework in which physicians and hospitals could alter some of their routine practices, without ever challenging the physician-patient relationship, or the notion that "normal" childbirth was fraught with potential pathology, even once the baby was born.

Most childbirth educators did not question either the male bias or the wide-ranging methodological deficits in the research studies. Rather, this research was seen by many as a validation of women's emotional and physical need to be close to their babies after birth, and helped normalize the feelings of alienation and isolation that resulted with routine separation. Penny Simkin, childbirth educator/author and major figure in the doula movement, recalls the impact of hearing about this research on childbirth educators:

> We had Marshall Klaus come to Seattle to speak in 1976 on bonding and the importance of mother-infant contact. It was a huge convention, over 1,300 people…He captured the love and respect and admiration and everything of the whole childbirth education movement, with his message—a message that we all, as mothers, knew. I knew how I ached for my child after birth. And to have that validated, and documented, was a thrill beyond belief. I remember he got such a thunderous, lengthy, standing ovation that I thought the church was going to collapse. And he was astounded by the reception he got (P. Simkin, personal communication, February 15, 2000).

Klaus and Kennell struck a chord among women whose emotional responses to being separated from their newborns had not been validated by other clinicians. Their research on mother-infant bonding had been overlooked within medical science, but garnered attention in the popular media. As Drs.

Klaus and Kennell further pursued this line of research, it took them in unexpected directions, connecting them to a group of women who had been profoundly moved by their findings. Childbirth educators who advocated the incorporation of humanistic childbirth support into medical settings saw these physicians as important and valuable allies.

Humanistic Childbirth Support—Doula as Labor Support Provider (1980-present)

Another birth story of the doula comes from the ongoing practice of women attending births, which was accelerated during the 1970s when the childbirth movement gained momentum from similar sorts of advocacy also underway in women's health, patient rights, and alternative medicine movements (Sullivan & Weitz, 1988). During this time, many birth activists, childbirth educators, partners, friends, and family members accompanied women during birth.[8] Different forms of labor support were tried out during the early phase of the natural-childbirth movement, when unmedicated birth was a major goal: the labor coach/partner, typically the husband; the *monitrice*, a Lamaze-trained nurse who accompanies women in labor and has some clinical responsibilities, such as checking blood pressure and fetal heart tones; and the childbirth assistant, usually an aspiring midwife.[9]

---

8 In response to consumer demand and legal battles, patients have the right to bring anyone with them into the hospital as long as their advocate does not get in the way of the delivery of medical care (Annas, 1989 [1975]).

9 The Association of Labor Assistants and Childbirth Educators (ALACE) is an organization that recognizes the explicit overlap between aspiring midwives and doulas, and offers an introduction to some clinical tasks, such as vaginal examinations, in its doula training workshops. In 2009, ALACE underwent a re-organization, splitting into two distinct organizations: toLabor, the birth doula/labor assistant branch, and The International Birth and Wellness Project, the childbirth education branch.

While there has been some analysis of these labor support roles in childbirth research, the role of the "community" doula has been neglected. Many women claimed they had been doulas before it was called that, "before it had a name." These were women who said they were always the one in their social network to attend the births of family members or friends, who had no special interest in midwifery or nursing, but "found themselves" going to births a lot.

Although childbirth educators had been attending births as coaches throughout the 1970s, mostly when fathers were unable or unwilling, they did not receive specialized labor support training or refer to themselves as doulas. By the 1980s a father's presence at labor and delivery was assumed; men were expected to attend childbirth classes and act as labor coaches (Berry, 1988; Leavitt, 2009; Simkin, 1992b). But many educators, while feeling honored and thrilled to be present at births, felt frustrated and uncertain about their role. It was clear to them that classroom preparation alone was not sufficient for educating women and their partners about the reality of unmedicated labor and birth. They soon realized that their presence during labor and birth could provide extra support for women who wanted "natural childbirth."

As childbirth educators were exploring the dimension of their "bedside" role at births, development in the patient rights advocacy movement helped define the terms by which a non-related family member might provide labor support: as a "patient advocate." The early 1980s saw the emergence of several patient rights organizations, and from the mid-1990s, organizations focused on the training and support of patient advocates. Several organizations and universities offer coursework, and even certificate programs, in patient or health advocacy. Patient advocates are empowered to act in accordance with the patient's wishes, as long as they do not get in the way of the ability to deliver medical care. In many ways, calls for reform in childbirth presaged and proved that consumer demands for changes in medical practice could and would be heard. Today many patient advocacy organizations emphasize the importance of becoming a good, i.e., critical, responsible, and informed consumer of healthcare as part of the emerging humanistic paradigm within medicine (Davis-Floyd, 2001; Earp, French, & Gilkey, 2008).

As previously noted, in 1980, the scientific evidence of the power of relationship-centered care within childbirth emerged out of the work of pediatricians Klaus and Kennell, and greatly influenced the development of the humanistic dimension of labor support—the doula. As these medical researchers pursued their interests in mother-infant bonding, they discovered and drew upon anthropologist Dana Raphael's concept of the doula, which she defined as an experienced mother helping new mothers, especially with breastfeeding assistance and support (Raphael, 1973). Klaus and Kennell, however, were interested in whether and how the timing of this role of "mothering the mother" would affect their primary research focus: which factors inhibit and enhance mother-infant bonding. They considered how to structure a study that would incorporate the "doula," and at what point in the process—two or six weeks postpartum, or during labor? Their decision to incorporate the doula as an independent variable during labor rather than postpartum led to their study of Guatemalan women: assessing whether the mother-infant relationship would benefit from the presence of a supportive lay woman (a "doula") throughout labor in an unsupportive and busy hospital environment (Sosa, Kennell, Robertson, & Urrutia, 1980).

This pilot study, along with subsequent trials in other locations, found that not only did mother-infant bonding increase, but in addition:

> The presence of a doula reduces the overall cesarean rate by 50 percent, length of labor by 25 percent, oxytocin use by 40 percent, pain medication by 30 percent, and the need for forceps by 40 percent, and requests for epidurals by 60 percent (Klaus, Kennell, & Klaus, 1993, p. 51).

Outcomes also improved in the control group, where an observer sat in the room taking notes. In answer to the question "What helped you most?" women in this group reportedly answered, "The woman that watched over me," referring to this observer.

Meta-analyses of these and 15 other randomized controlled trials have confirmed the substance of these early findings, if to varying degrees (Hodnett, 1999; Hodnett, Gates, Hofmeyr, & Sakala, 2012; Hodnett, Stremler, Willan, Weston, Lowe, Simpson, . . . Gafni, 2009). Studies among middle-class patients at hospitals owned and operated by health management organizations have not found such dramatic benefits, especially in terms of operative deliveries (and the associated cost savings), but the emotional benefits to birthing women were still found to be significant (Gordon, Walton, McAdam, Derman, Gallitero, & Garrett, 1999). One observer (Richards, 1992) notes that these early trials took place in hospitals where the majority of women were of very low socioeconomic status and not permitted to have anyone with them. Richards concludes: " ... perhaps what the presence of a doula did was to improve the quality and appropriateness of staff actions toward the laboring woman" (Richards, 1992, p. 41).

Another response to a study that found little change in the birth outcomes of women attended by a professional *monitrice* was that the early clinical trials adopted obstetric practice protocols in order to control for variation in individual physician practice, especially with regard to the cesarean decision (Hodnett & Osborn, 1989a; Shearer, 1989). The fact that laboring women in the control group of the early clinical trials also experienced better maternal/neonatal outcomes supports this interpretation—and allows us to make sense of more recent studies conducted among middle-class populations where no significant differences were found in medical interventions or outcomes.

Feminist critiques of research about mother-infant bonding focus on its ideological underpinnings, placing women's relationships with their babies onto a feminist battleground encompassing women's roles in private and public social worlds. "Bonding theory is prejudiced against women pursuing a life in which children are not the *raison d'etre* of women or their exclusive focus of attention" (Arney, 1980, p. 173). Arney explains why placing women's emotions at the center of obstetric practice would destabilize the power of obstetrics, and how bonding theory protects against this.

> Admitting women's subjectivity to the discourse about obstetrics would be disconcerting. A theory, the embodiment of objectivity, can be used as the basis for a response to the concerns of women without allowing the subjective, passionate component to surface and disrupt obstetrical work. Bonding is a theory which allowed obstetrics to change in order to keep the social relations, on which its work was based, the same in the calls for fundamental reform. The disorder which women threatened to bring to the profession was prevented by reworking the old order and adapting it to a new situation (Arney, 1980, p. 174).

And yet, admitting women's subjectivity to feminist critiques can also be disconcerting. Doulas are aware and critical of the social control mechanisms that obstetrics wields over women, even if they do not see this in the ideological context of bonding and its connection to the doula research. However, they strategically used the power of scientific validation to advance their own women-centered agendas. A doula in my study, Rose Peters, understood that Klaus and Kennell's research was not about women, nor based on experience providing labor support:

> Now, they're pedies [pediatricians], and they came into this research about the babies. It didn't have anything to do about the mothers. And so they really didn't know

what they were looking for other than what was making a difference to the baby. And to this day, they've never done any of the work, everybody's like "this is wonderful, this is the stuff, these people did this, et cetera." No, neither one of those nice men ever did this. [INT: You mean labor support...] Exactly. I don't think they've even been there to a whole birth (Rose Peters).

Such critiques notwithstanding, many childbirth educators embraced Klaus and Kennell's research and used the early Guatemala study, as well as subsequent trials, to convince women, and more importantly, their obstetricians, of the importance of labor support provided by a non-family member.

Not all feminist scholars are skeptical of the research claims with regard to the labor support role. Historian Judith Walzer Leavitt notes the early clinical trial research in the epilogue of her book on childbearing in America from 1750-1950.

Perhaps even more exciting, within the context of what we have learned from history, recent research by Marshall Klaus, John Kennell, and their colleagues reveals that the presence of a supportive person during labor and delivery significantly shortens labor and may reduce complications ... Women who have argued that they need to bring into the hospital people whom they can rely upon—women, in other words, who seek to repeat the collective experience of their foremothers—find that controlled research is reinforcing their position by showing that such support improves the course and outcome of labor. The age-old practice of cooperative behavior around the birthing bed has found a modern day scientific reason for its long-lasting practices; women's traditions are finding their way into medical hospital-based obstetrics (Leavitt, 1986, p. 217).

The phrase "women's traditions were finding their way into medical hospital-based obstetrics" overlooks just how this was accomplished. The articulation of the "doula as professional labor support" encompassed years of work as several women—together and individually—developed, elaborated, and communicated the particular way "traditions" would or could be adapted to "modern" childbirth support. While individual women (and childbirth educators) in community networks were attending births as soon as hospitals permitted a support person, the first organized labor support course was offered at The Birth Place in Menlo Park, California.

The Birth Place was an independent birth resource center and freestanding birth center co-founded in 1979 by childbirth activist Suzanne Arms and obstetrician Don Creevy, among others. From the start, the notion of labor support was integral to the founders' goal of achieving out-of-hospital childbirth, influenced by the writings of Dick-Read, Bradley, and Lamaze. In addition, Suzanne Arms knew Klaus and Kennell, and was familiar with their research on bonding and the two Guatemala studies. Indeed, Joan Barbour, director of The Birth Place from 1979 through 1982, recalls that the "doula" training began sometime early on in her tenure, and found a copy of the 1980 doula research article in her files (Sosa, Kennell, Robertson, & Urrutia, 1980). Barbour remembers using the term "doula" to refer to this position in her presentations to potential clients. The doula was described in these presentations as:

> … a non-medically trained person there to help women and their families by doing things that a midwife, doctor, or nurse would not be doing, such as applying cool washcloths, doing massage, cooking, looking after children—anything to make the woman and her family comfortable (J. Barbour, personal communication, April 27, 2002).

The doula trainings were loosely organized, perhaps offered about twice a year, with various speakers. Suzanne Arms remembers teaching some of the classes and bringing in others to teach as well:

These classes were taught by various people in the community who had different skills and perspectives to bring: from the beginning we had incorporated mind, body, spirit, as well as political issues and the history of birthing, all of which we felt were important for doulas to understand along with hands-on care. I know I gave several classes (S. Arms, personal communication, May 3, 2002).

Henci Goer, who attended doula training at The Birth Place, recalled some of the early debates about the definition and scope of the labor support role (H. Goer, personal communication, January 3, 2002). There were ongoing debates among those who thought clinical skills, such as monitoring fetal heart rates or checking cervical dilation, should be part of the labor support role. Another issue was whether the doula should be a volunteer service rather than a paid profession. Goer felt The Birth Place vision of the doula as a volunteer contributed to the large turnover among the growing number of doulas who were being trained, and recalls at the time: "I defined that as a problem. I chose the philosophical position that this was professional work and should be compensated" (H. Goer, personal communication, January 3, 2002).

Goer described two main types of women who came to these early trainings but did not continue in the field as doulas: women who were initially enthusiastic about going to births, but found the work difficult to manage with other demands (small children) in their lives and became rapidly burned out; and women who were aspiring midwives who obtained the necessary labor support training and experience through the doula work, then moved on to midwifery practice. Either way, the challenge for the Birth Place and these early doula trainers was to identify and support a group of women who could continue to do this work over the long run.

The Birth Place closed its doors in 1994, after malpractice issues of the mid-1980s caused it to transition to a proprietary center directed by a nurse-midwife and physician Don Creevy (J. Barbour, personal communication, April 27, 2002). However, the shift in organizational structure had resulted in the loss of the extensive resource center and allied training programs. To fill this gap, an early Birth Place trainee and Bradley childbirth educator, Claudia Lowe, began to further elaborate and specify the role of labor support provider. In 1983, she founded the Association of Childbirth Assistants as a local support group. Lowe remembered hearing from women all over the country who expressed great interest in labor support training, which led her to expand the organization the next year, as the National Association of Childbirth Assistants (NACA) (C. Lowe, personal communication, January 24, 2002).

From 1984 to 1994, under Lowe's leadership, NACA held childbirth assistant trainings across the country, and published a newsletter. In 1990, Lowe self-published a book in loose-leaf format, entitled *Becoming a Childbirth Assistant: The Lowe Method.* This book encapsulates much of what was being substantively offered in the NACA trainings and became a supplement to more interactive and role-playing activities as the trainings were refined (C. Lowe, personal communication, January 24, 2002).

Concerned about the variety of terms being used to designate labor support or assistance and worried about using a term that lacked a distinctive focus for labor support, Lowe provided a glossary to distinguish between the terms commonly in use. "Childbirth assistant," according to Lowe, described someone who provides a comprehensive service of labor support and educational counseling for the childbearing year. Highlights in this role were extensive prenatal and postpartum client visits in addition to the birth itself, as Lowe wrote in her manual.

Additional factors that make this caregiver so distinct is consumer advocacy by the client before the labor and birth experience (client-directed consumer advocacy), postpartum planning, optimum support techniques, social support systems, individualized care, statement of disclosure and "planning your day of labor" (Lowe, 1990/1992, p. 17).

The terminology defined the childbirth assistant role as extending from pregnancy to postpartum, versus focusing on one point in this continuum. For example, Lowe saw Labor Support Persons or Labor Support Professionals as present during labor and birth only, with limited pre- and post-natal contact. Doulas, following Dana Raphael's definition, were those who provided postpartum home care or home help along the lines of Postpartum Assistants.

Lowe's practical reasoning and personal experience in the best way to provide labor support became one of the first formally articulated descriptions of the childbirth assistant, although her book was never widely distributed. On the issue of medical vs. non-medical skills for the Childbirth Assistant (CA), Lowe advocated non-medical skills as sufficient.

In our role as Childbirth Assistants, we believe non-medical care and support can provide effective and long-term benefits. We feel it can preserve the art of labor support and the ability to care for women using the intuitive arts of active listening, intuition, counseling, and friending, among others (Lowe, 1990/1992, p. 72).

Furthermore, she notes:

Use of medical skills can interfere with a woman's ability to look within herself for signs of labor and birth. It provides a false measurement for the Childbirth Assistant and prevents her from observing and knowing the signs of labor and birth. If we propose to trust women, their innate abilities and birth itself, then we must demonstrate that belief in our actions toward the women we serve (p. 72).

Recognizing that many Childbirth Assistants believe in a certain model of birth as "best," Lowe addressed a dilemma that remains an issue in doula practice today: how to support a woman who is choosing interventions that the doula considers unnecessary or harmful.

Her birth is her birth. It is not a birth that her Childbirth Assistant believes is right ... As Childbirth Assistants, the Lowe Method encourages us to stop telling women how they should give birth and start listening to how they want to give birth (p. 4).

Lowe was one of the original doula trainers who stressed the importance of clarifying these two issues: the childbirth assistant is a non-medically trained support person who validates women's own choices regarding their own births.[10]

At its height, NACA organizational membership included about 300 certified childbirth assistants, and Lowe estimated she and others trained over 1,000 women in their ten-year history. Lowe also founded Birth Support Providers International, which she intended to be an umbrella organization for the various doula organizations coming into existence, but this effort did not receive widespread support. Although engaged in early discussions with the eventual founders of Doulas of North America/DONA International, the two groups did not have any formal association. After a decade of running NACA and contributing greatly to the understanding of the labor support role, Lowe ended her organizational involvement in 1994. (C. Lowe, personal communication, January 24, 2002). One of Lowe's former students says, "Claudia got people to

---

10 See also (Perez, 1990/1994).

think globally" about the role of labor support (M. Jackson, personal communication, January 23, 2002).

This global role for labor support found a growing audience in the ranks of childbirth educators, who were the new front line of women with direct contact with childbearing women, prenatally and postpartum. As childbirth education gained in numbers and professional status, its organizations began to sponsor seminars to educate members about research on childbirth experiences. These professionals were uniquely poised to not only observe, but to act upon their intuition and information about what women wanted and needed during birth. The Klaus and Kennell research findings on the impact of continuous labor support for women's emotional satisfaction with birth reinforced what many childbirth educators, and doulas already knew.

> I didn't know about their research stuff, nor did I want to. But I did see how it was going to interface with my work with women. [INT: How did you see that it would?] Well, because of their name, you know, anything in this OB [obstetric] or medical world has got to have a male doctor's name on it. So if I could use their name to get what I needed done for the women in my area that was fine with me. (Rose Peters).

In this context, two childbirth educators—one a nurse, the other a physical therapist—devoted their careers to defining the role of the professional labor support person, or doula: Paulina (Polly) Perez and Penny Simkin. Recounting how she saw the doula come into existence, Simkin noted:

> So we had Klaus and Kennell's research, we had my own research, and the fact that I'd been at births and people telling me what a difference I'd made. We'd had

Claudia Lowe, and we had the *monitrice*.[11] There were all these little fragments (P. Simkin, personal communication, February 15, 2000).

Putting these fragments together created a phenomenon. According to Penny Simkin, hundreds of childbirth educators were exploring a more direct role during labor and birth in the late 1970s and early 1980s. Whether asked by their childbirth education students to attend the birth, or volunteering for family and friends, many women who were birth activists during this time period described a variation on the theme: "I was a doula before they called it that." Many childbirth educators knew about the dramatic findings of improved birth outcomes with a doula present because they had been following the bonding research of Drs. Klaus and Kennell. Birth activists were not greatly surprised by the findings, but were pleased to have scientific evidence to support their own growing experience and knowledge of the value of labor support. During this time, the name and definition and practical scope of this newly "rediscovered" labor support role received attention from many people across the country, with these two childbirth educators providing a public face for labor support through publishing, training, and organizational development. While Simkin preferred the term "professional labor support person" and Perez refers to the "professional labor assistant" in her book, the term "doula" was associated with the research of Klaus and Kennell. Soon, "doula" become the agreed-upon term for the role, and was incorporated in the organizational name Doulas of North America in 1992.

Polly Perez

Like several other nurses in the early 1970s, Paulina (Polly) Perez worked as a nurse-*monitrice*, a licensed or registered

11 Referring to the Lamaze tradition in general, and Polly Perez, in particular.

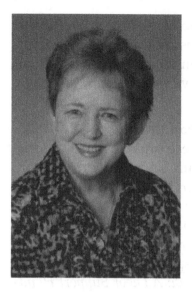

Photo 8: Paulina (Polly) Perez, an internationally known author, perinatal nurse and lecturer, whose early work championed the labor support role.
Photo provided by Polly Perez.

nurse trained in Lamaze method of natural childbirth. Nurse-*monitrices* typically taught childbirth education classes at hospitals where they were employed. The nurse-*monitrice* differs from the doula or labor support person in that she incorporates medical assessment, such as cervical dilation, into her role. An early pioneer in this role in the U.S., Polly Perez recalls her travels across the country "giving speeches to nurses about OB [obstetric] things, nothing about doulas." At these talks, she was introduced as a *monitrice*, and nurses would approach her afterward and want to know what that was, what she did, and how she did it. She recalled, "I got so many questions, I decided to write a book." At the time, she says, 'the only thing in print was a little booklet on *monitrices* that was published in the 1970s, but gone by the 1980s."

Beginning in the mid-1980s, Perez interviewed women who were providing labor support. Published in 1990, *Special Women* was the first book that examined the work of professional labor assistants, as she called them, highlighting the emotional as well as the practical dimensions of the role. The book was geared primarily toward aspiring doulas and included chapters on how to set up a professional practice, how to foster effective communications and relationships with obstetric clinicians, and information about psychological and medical issues in pregnancy. One chapter contained personal memories from women who had had labor assistants at their births, and another chapter highlighted three perspectives from physicians on the role of labor assistants. This book linked the growing community of obstetric nurses, childbirth educators, and labor support professionals by emphasizing their common goal—increasing women's emotional satisfaction with their birth experiences—while differentiating their diverse roles and responsibilities.

Perez founded Childbirth and Family Education in 1990, and Cutting Edge Press in 1994. These organizations are still in existence. Perez continues to lecture and write on the topic of labor support and to offer doula trainings. She has been on the board of advisors for Childbirth and Postpartum Professionals Association (CAPPA) since its inception in 1998. Perez's business is largely centered around products and books for childbirth professionals, with a special emphasis on labor assistants. *The Nurturing Touch at Birth: A Labor Support Handbook* was published in 1997. This book, geared toward professional labor assistants, nurses, and others working with laboring women, focuses on specific techniques and positions for easing labor pain and enhancing labor progress.

Penny Simkin

Another pioneer in doula organizational history and role definition has been childbirth educator and author Penny Simkin. As she recounts her journey, Simkin began accompanying her childbirth students to their births around 1968, but without a clear sense of her role at the birth itself. She tells a story about a birth that galvanized her thinking about the labor support role. Sometime in the mid-1970s, Simkin was invited for the labor of one of her childbirth education students.

I was thrilled. There was no talk about what I would do; I didn't think I'd do anything. So I was there standing against the wall, and admiring this whole thing, and I'll never forget some of the wonderful things that hap-

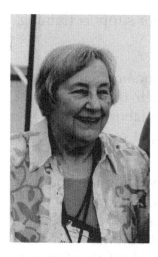

Photo 9: Penny Simkin at the 2012 DONA International Conference in Cancun, Mexico. A pioneer in the field, she remains active in her mid-70s.

Photo by Kyndal May.

pened during that labor. They had a four-year-old there, she was lying on the bed, just about four feet from the woman's perineum, just rapt, and after the baby was born, she insisted that the baby be called Rosie. But later, when we talked about it, the mother asked, "Why didn't you say anything?" I said, "Well, I didn't want to interrupt, or disturb you." I thought I should be definitely on the outskirts. And she said, "I thought you disapproved." And I felt horrible. I had been with women who I had helped, but these were needy single women, or ones where we'd planned that they needed some help. I was shaken by that [the woman's sense that Penny had disapproved]. Here I was, full of admiration for her, I was feeling so honored to be there, and she was thinking I was disapproving. That shook me, terribly. And I realized if I'm going to be there, I'm going to do something.

After this experience, Simkin began exploring both the role and the experiences of others similarly engaged. She said she knew she was on to something big when she offered a Sharing Circle on Labor Support at an International Childbirth Education Association (ICEA) conference in 1987, and over 100 women showed up. She recalls:

It was a mob scene ... and from that we came up with a newsletter, just to bind people together who were interested, and I did that three times [over the next few years]. There was a huge interest, I tried to get ICEA to sponsor a doula training, we were calling it labor support training, but they wouldn't do it.

Despite the lack of institutional sponsorship, Simkin used her ICEA connections (she'd been on their board for several years) to spread the word about the labor support role through her newsletter and by speaking at conferences and workshops.

Her first efforts were local: after convincing the board of directors of the Seattle Midwifery School, Simkin offered her first labor support training under its auspices in 1988. After this training, the class members met with Simkin to form a local support group, the Pacific Association for Labor Support (PALS). The initial purpose of the organization was to provide moral support for each other as they waited for clients. As time went on, the members took steps to incorporate the organization and establish by-laws, standards of practice, and a code of ethics.

Simkin had a wealth of information on labor support and published *The Birth Partner* in 1989. This book articulated a birth companion role, assumed in most cases to be the father of the baby, not necessarily a doula, or even a woman. In the book, now in its fourth edition, Simkin refers to a professional labor support person:

> … who has perspective and experience. A labor support person can raise your morale and the mother's, make concrete suggestions for comfort measures, help you remember some of the things you learned in childbirth class, and remind you and the mother of her Birth Plan. With the unfamiliarity and stress of labor, you might welcome an experienced, calm advocate who can remain with you through the birth (Simkin, 1989/2013, p. 92).

Despite her strong influence on the development and growth of the doula role and doula organizations, Simkin devotes relatively little space to doulas in her published books. This stands in contrast to her extensive physical and intellectual contributions. Simkin profoundly shaped the organizational definition of the doula in the early days of PALS and DONA International. She has conducted hundreds of trainings and special workshops, continuing into her 70s. She was instrumental in the development of training curricula and certification guidelines, and authored scores of handouts that are included in doula training notebooks. Her ongoing personal experience of attending births as a doula has been a source of experiential knowledge that she has used in her organizational work. She told me from her home office in Seattle, "My own personal journey, a lot of it has been reflected in the evolution of douladom, here—anyway" (P. Simkin, personal communication, February 15, 2000). Simkin played a crucial role in the founding of Doulas of North America, along with Annie Kennedy, then president of the Pacific Association for Labor Support, and Marshall Klaus, MD, Phyllis Klaus, MSW, and John Kennell, MD, in 1992.[12]

As two of the first writers to articulate the experience of childbirth educators and nurses in providing labor support, Penny Simkin and Polly Perez conveyed the power and potential of an emotionally satisfying birth experience. They also observed and wrote about the effects of a disempowering, emotionally traumatic birth experience on women's postpartum adjustment. Both Simkin and Perez were vocal advocates for how labor support would help women have an emotionally satisfying birth. Their work clearly shows the limited, partial story conveyed by clinical trials claiming medical benefits to labor support.

---

12 In 2004, Doulas of North America (DONA) officially changed its name to DONA International, to reflect the growing membership in countries outside North America.

Simkin was inspired by what she learned when women's emotional concerns were placed at the center of labor support practice. In the early 1990s, she embarked on a research project, the findings of which would eventually become a cornerstone of doula training: validating the reality that women retain emotional memories of their birth experience. Prior to this research, Simkin was questioning her future, and uncertain about the impact of her work as a childbirth educator. She shares her story of how she took up this research project and the moral she derived from its findings.

For me personally, when I realized that birth matters, and how a woman gives birth is with her for the rest of her life—the story that got me even thinking about this research was from an old woman. I was teaching in the cafeteria of a convalescent center, and this 84-year-old woman came into my class, and she'd sit in the back and stay there. And it was hot in there, with these poor swollen pregnant women, all red faced with veins popping out—because they kept it about 80 degrees—and here was this woman in her robe and paper slippers in the back. After about the fourth class, she raised her hand, and it just threw me. I was the only one who could see her, because everybody was facing me and she was in the back, and I said, "Yes … " She thought she was in a class, and she stood up and said, "I had three babies," and she started reciting all the details, and I thought, "My god, this woman is 84 and she remembers her births! She probably can't remember what she ate tonight for dinner," and I thought, "Gosh, this is important." That's what really clicked, that's when I decided I had something to offer here. (P. Simkin, personal communication, February 15, 2000).

In the research inspired by this woman's story, Simkin contacted women from her childbirth classes who had given birth to their first child between 1968 and 1974. She asked them to fill out a birth questionnaire and write down their birth story, some 15 to 20 years after their births. Simkin then compared these stories with the ones the women had given to her right after their births, and which they hadn't seen in the interim (long before the days of photocopies and birth stories on the web) (Simkin, 1991, 1992a). Her personal investment in this study stemmed from having second thoughts about whether any of her hard work in childbirth was "worth it." She found her life's mission and passion in the answer.

> I did my study of long-term birth memories, and as I was doing that, I realized the ingredient as to whether the woman felt satisfied or not was not pain, complications, length of labor, or any of those things, but how she felt she was cared for. Really, that gelled it for me. I mean, I made a vow: I'm going to do everything in my power to make sure every woman who has a baby is well cared for. The moving stories some of those women told me … I was crying with some of them. I just can't tell you what a huge impact that had on me. (P. Simkin, personal communication, February 15, 2000).

This study has had a central place in doula training ever since its publication. It validated and underscored the emotional significance of labor and birth throughout women's lives, not just in the short term. Echoing Kitzinger's sentiment, then, but in less erotic terms, Simkin places women's satisfaction with their birth at the center of her understanding of the doula role. Simkin's research focused not on medical outcomes as a great benefit of doula care, but on women feeling like they were at the center of the drama of their own birth experiences. Simkin shifted the focus from the interventions (or the lack thereof) to the women themselves. As one early doula trainer, Kris Turner noted, "It was kind of a wake-up call when she finished that—Oh, it's not just about natural birth."

With the medicalization of childbirth support firmly entrenched, the idea of turning labor support into a specialized service niche that would complement but not overtly threaten or question ongoing medical management of childbirth support proved to be successful in attracting women who wished to provide this type of support, as well as women who wished to receive it. Its roots in the natural childbirth movement, the doula movement, like La Leche League (LLL), formed early and cooperative liaisons with physicians (Ward, 2000). Again, like LLL, the early founders and elaborators of doula care tapped into the relevance of women's experience as central to their mission, drawing on research from male physicians that provided scientific legitimization for viewing this experience as consequential for women's and their babies' health.

Doula Organizations and Terminology

One of Simkin's original goals in founding Doulas of North America (DONA) was to create an umbrella organization that would approve training curricula and certification programs of labor support organizations around the country. Although several childbirth organizations have now included labor support training as part of their offerings, most did not gather under DONA's umbrella. NACA did not merge with DONA, and subsequently disbanded as an organization in late 1994. After DONA's emergence in 1992, existing national childbirth education organizations, such as the Association of Labor Assistants and Childbirth Educators (ALACE) in 1995, International Childbirth Education Association (ICEA) in 1996, and BirthWorks in 1999, developed programs to train and certify doulas. Before these programs, ALACE and BirthWorks had been incorporating labor support within their childbirth education training.

Other organizations formed as an alternative to DONA's vision and version of labor support, including Childbirth and Postpartum Professionals Association (CAPPA) in 1998. CAPPA became the first organization to offer three types of training and certification (labor support, postpartum support, and childbirth education) and include distance-learning program options. Eventually CAPPA added lactation support and other training and certification options. Over the past 20 years, a fast-growing industry of doula training workshops, offered by local trainers affiliated with numerous certifying organizations espousing diverse birth philosophies, has emerged in the United States.

One obvious point of difference for organizations has been around terminology: what to call the person who provides labor support. The term doula was used by the Birth Place to describe the work of labor support, as early as 1979 to 1980. DONA International has made the word "doula" a more recognizable one by its large membership and public relations efforts. Yet other organizations have chosen alternative descriptors they feel better represent their underlying philosophy on the labor support role, including Birth Guide, Birth Doula, Holistic Doula, Labor Assistant, Labor Doula, Labor Support Specialist, Childbirth Assistant, and Birth Support Practitioner. ALACE (now called toLabor, as of 2009) provides the only case of an organization consciously choosing to NOT use the term doula due to its connotations to slavery and women's subordination in the original Greek context (J. Porter, personal communication, January 23, 2002).

Many attribute the near-universal adoption of the term "doula" to Marshall Klaus' advocacy during the formation of Doulas of North America (DONA). One doula, Rose Peters, recounts early discussions with the DONA founders in which she promoted the view that "doula is really about postpartum. But he [Marshall Klaus] was so attached to that word and wouldn't let it go." In the Seattle area, the term doula was not well known, or even desired, in the early 1990s. "We didn't even call ourselves doulas, you know, until we sort of felt forced to, we were labor support people" (P. Simkin, personal communication, February 15, 2000). Seattle-area doula trainer Kris Turner offers her perspective: "For the first couple of years, we resisted calling ourselves doulas. We called ourselves labor support, but we decided that using the word doula gives us a chance to educate people about what we do."

The extent to which terminology implies a difference in perspective or emphasis in how labor support is provided/what it entails is an empirical question. While nearly all organizations that train and certify doulas acknowledge a bias toward natural (unmedicated, low-to-non-interventive) childbirth, they nevertheless also state in their written materials that it is up to birthing women to choose the kind of birth they want. Some organizations, like Birth Works and Birthing From Within, place more emphasis on the emotional and spiritual aspects of the birth experience—for the woman, the baby, and the father, as well as the doula. Some organizations take the position that doulas are not required for a good birth experience—that doulas can also be seen as an intervention into the "natural" process of birth. Additional research needs to be done on how various organizations orient toward the role of the doula and their underlying perception of birth to address these issues.

The alternative birth community, of which the doula is a part (despite the aspirations of doulas to be mainstream) remains highly diversified in an organizational sense, even if not as diverse in philosophies about birth and policies about the labor support role. The multiplicity of doula training organizations today reflects ideological and interpersonal tensions operating at the grassroots level as well as organizational competition for market share for aspiring doulas and pregnant clients. Without a national registry, it is nearly impossible to account for the number of doula-training workshops, the number of women trained and certified as doulas, or how many actively practicing doulas exist in the United States today.

Social Context of the Emergence of Doulas in the United States

Doulas emerged as a viable, humanistic labor support role in a social context that saw the rise of women's health advocacy and patient rights' movements, midwifery, and alternative medicine; and most recently the Internet. Doulas eagerly adapted technology to disseminate their perspectives and, perhaps most relevant, connect with each other since the Internet exploded into public consciousness in the mid-1990s. Through websites, YouTube, and social networking sites, the Internet has exponentially added to the availability of women's experiences with and information about pregnancy and birth. As early as 2001, web search engine results for the word "doula" produced 55,200 "hits" using Google, and 30,600 web pages (47 websites) using Yahoo! (In 2010, there were over 440,000 hits on Google, and by 2013, 5,310,000).[13] Doulas are standard mentions in every one of the numerous websites that devote extensive resources to information and discussion boards on pregnancy and childbirth topics.

Doulas themselves use the Internet to communicate with each other and with their client base through online discussion boards, and social networking sites. The growth of online networks is visible in the rise in the number of Yahoo! Groups over a decade. In August 2001, there were about 50 Yahoo!

---

13 As a comparison, a Google.com search on the word "midwife" produced 238,000 results (search 10/17/01) and 11,800,000 (search 5/26/13), while the word "obstetrician" produced about 65,200 results (search 10/17/01) and 8,030,000 (search 5/26/13). Yahoo search results on "midwife" found 90,000 web pages/162 websites, and "obstetrician" found 40,200 web pages/20 websites in a search done on 10/17/01.

Groups containing the word "doula," and just ten years later, there were 1,077 Yahoo! Groups. In addition to public and private discussion boards, doulas construct a vibrant web presence through individual and organizational websites, blogs, videos, and fan pages on social networking sites.

The constellation of these cultural, technological, and social factors intersected in the mid-1980s through the late-1990s to provide a synergistic environment for the emergence and growing public acceptance of the labor support role. At the same time, there was a growing interest in humanistic model of medicine in the United States:

Humanism arose in reaction to [the excesses of technomedicine] as an effort driven by nurses and physicians working within the medical system to reform it from the inside. Humanists wish simply to humanize technomedicine—that is, to make it relational, partnership-oriented, individually responsive, and compassionate. This caring, common-sensical approach is garnering wide international appreciation and support (Davis-Floyd, 2002, p. S5).

Doulas, as embodiment of the humanistic element of supportive care within childbirth, have the potential to "open the technocratic system, from the inside, to the possibility of widespread reform" (Davis-Floyd, 2002, p. S5). However, due to the specific contours and dilemmas embedded within the role, doula care has the potential to be co-opted by technocratic medicine in much the same way as childbirth education has been.

The Doula as a Uniquely American Response to Changing Maternity Care

The changes in pain management, obstetric technology, and professional roles in maternity care over the past 100 years have created a unique space for the doula role. Pregnant women are bombarded with information, advice, and stories about childbirth from many directions. Much of this advice is conflicting and places the pregnant woman in the midst of ongoing debates over the safety of medical interventions, the meaning of pain, and the best way to have a baby in the United States (Klassen, 2001; Michie & Cahn, 1997; Pincus, 2000). Even the educated, middle-class woman with many resources can find all of this overwhelming, and feel let down and betrayed by the medical system of care for pregnant women (Block, 2007; Wolf, 2001). Childbirth advocates have long argued that obstetric practice does not follow scientific research to ensure optimal maternal and neonatal outcomes (Enkin, Keirse, Neilson, Crowther, Duley, Hodnett, & Hofmeyr, 2000; Goer, 1995; Goer & Romano, 2012; Sakala & Corry, 2008).

Amidst the cacophony of advice and information surrounding pregnancy and childbirth, the doula emerged in the U.S. as both a consumerist and woman-centered response to the need for emotional and informational support during this significant life transition. The doula has been a uniquely American response to this dilemma, as a British physician addressing this issue noted.

> If nobody can fill this [labor support] role, or the available people are denied access to the hospital, what should be done? From a European perspective, the answer seems obvious—provide continuity of care from an appropriately trained midwife and pressure the hospital until it makes humane arrangements for delivery so that any mother can have whoever she chooses with her during labor and birth (Richards, 1992, p. 41).

However, the proportion of all U.S. births attended by certified nurse-midwives (CNMs), while increasing from 3.3% of all births in 1989 to a high of 7.7% of all births in 2002, has remained fairly steady according to the most recent data available: 7.6% in 2009 (Declercq, 2012). In a maternity context, with so few midwife-attended births in the late 1980s and early 1990s, childbirth educators endeavored to fill the emotional gap in U.S. maternity care by forming organizations to train and certify labor support doulas and articulating the need for emotional support in childbirth.

Today, in training workshops and in marketing their services, doulas portray their role in maternity care within a historical framework that highlights the universality and particularity of woman-to-woman support during childbirth. This historical framework claims the universality of emotional care during birth, yet poses significant challenges for doulas as they endeavor to accomplish that care in the current context of childbearing in the United States.

While much research underscores the nature and importance of social support during childbirth, it is not clear whether the doula, as an intermediary between the woman's emotional experience of her birth and the medical management of it, has a significant role to play in addressing larger systemic change in U.S. maternity care. Can doulas, as non-medically-trained outsiders to the hospital, effectively reverse rising cesarean rates and worsening maternal health outcomes? Are doulas a mere bandage on a hemorrhage, softening the effects of institutional childbirth, because they do not overtly challenge medical authority over normal birth, thus supporting the status quo (Morton & Basile, 2013; Simonds, Rothman & Norman, 2006)?

Alternatively, are doulas, given their online visibility, the grassroots nature and relative accessibility of their training workshops, and ideological alignment with the midwifery model of care, able to raise awareness of, and consequently, consumer demand for midwifery care in the United States? Will the growing interest in developing community-based doula programs within Medicaid expand availability of continuous labor support to women of lower socioeconomic status? Can a model of emotional support in labor, based largely on the experiences of middle-class white women, be relevant to all women giving birth in the United States today? The answers to these complex questions are found within larger cultural debates over the "good birth," safe and healthy outcomes, the role of technology and obstetric authority, and women's bodies and roles as mothers, and are considered throughout this book.

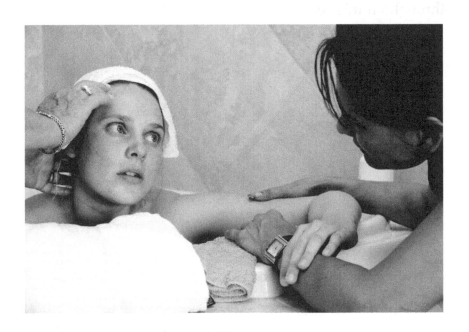

Photo 10. The doula's emotional connection to her client is made through direct eye contact and nurturing touch with the laboring woman. *Photo by Kyndal May.*

Personal Story

DOULAS REALLY MAKE A DIFFERENCE
Ellen Derby

I gave birth to my first daughter in 1992. It was not a long birth by many standards, and it was natural. I was healthy and so was my daughter. I was attended by a midwife, and my mother was there, along with my baby's father. Still, it was not the birth I wanted. My daughter was traumatized, breast-feeding was a problem, and I spent too much time alone. I was disillusioned and aggrieved.

Labor started nicely at 9:00 p.m., and in my mind, progressed well. I called my midwife when the contractions were a minute long and five minutes apart. She said to come into the hospital for a check. She said my uterus was "nervous," gave me a sleeping pill, and sent me home, saying to come back as much as I wanted.

Back home in bed, I had a difficult contraction. My child's father was sound asleep, and I felt alone. Since he wasn't much help or comfort while awake, I didn't bother waking him. Instead, I labored quietly resting on the couch, taking a bath, visualizing, telling myself I could do this. I could handle being alone, but it was hard to draw the bath, get in and out of the tub, and dress myself. I would have been calmer and more comforted if someone had been with me. A warm touch, a smile, and kind words would have made the experience so much nicer.

By early morning my legs were shaking, and I was having trouble staying on top of contractions. I woke my partner and impressed upon him the need to get moving. I called the midwives, got dressed, and made it down three flights of stairs.

In the hospital room, I learned to my dismay that my midwife was not there. I was put in a traditional labor room instead of the labor-delivery-recovery room I had expected. I continued to struggle with contractions, and told the nurse I might want something to help. She said, "It's too late for that now."

I felt like I might have to push, and the midwife on call wasn't there yet. A doctor I'd never seen before was told to check me. He was very kind. I was in transition at nine centimeters.

Finally, the midwife arrived. My mother got there a little later. The midwife said I could push. My waters still hadn't broken. The midwife told me it would help the baby come faster if she broke them, so I acquiesced. Because there was some meconium, I had to go to the delivery room. That was when my birth turned emotionally traumatic.

The delivery room was cold, the table hard. A nurse stood in the background. I clung to my mother. I felt the midwife was rushing me. She told me not to scream. It took about an hour to birth Elizabeth. Because the midwife was concerned about the meconium, she showed me my daughter briefly, and then took her to a little room next door where they deep suctioned her lungs.

In contrast, my last child was born in 2004. This was a short, intense, natural homebirth. Both of us were healthy. My mother, husband, and daughters were there, along with two friends. I had a new midwife and a doula. By then I had become a doula myself.

This was the best birth! It was peaceful and full of love. I was comfortable, comforted, and surrounded by caring people.

My labor began in the morning while I was sleeping. I roused every fifteen minutes for an hour or two before fully waking. I had a bloody show, so I was excited that today would be the day! I called my midwife, Sue, my doula, Mary Ann, my mom, and my friend Laurel to let them know.

Mary Ann stayed in touch during early labor. She kept encouraging me that soon I'd have my baby. While my mother and older daughter watched my four-year old, my husband and I went for a walk. Then we went to our room to cuddle and do some nipple stimulation to see if we could get the contractions moving. It worked. I called Mary Ann and Sue. My husband called Laurel, a doula and mother of eight. She hugged me and helped my mom and husband get things ready.

Soon Mary Ann was there. I was so happy to see her! Then Sue arrived. Mary Ann offered sips of water, held my back as I squatted, told me how great I was doing. When contractions were rough, she whispered words of encouragement while the midwife offered good suggestions. My husband made supper for my girls. Laurel smiled as she watched over me and prayed quietly. She offered cool cloths and water. There were five people in my bathroom, but it didn't feel crowded; it felt full of love.

I had another contraction, and as I pushed mightily, the baby slid out on a gush of water. My husband was on the bed with me, Mary Ann was nearby, and the others were in a circle around the bed. They held Katrina up through my legs. I held my beautiful daughter, as she gave a lusty cry in my arms. Everyone was emotional. I got lots of kisses and hugs from everyone.

Mary Ann fixed food. My husband hugged me while Sue sewed the three stitches I needed. I nursed my daughter peacefully. After a while, Sue and Laurel left. Mary Ann stayed with me until we were ready for her to go.

Having a doula made a huge difference in how I experienced birth. I was never alone. My doula's confidence and her belief in my body, my spirit, and my ability to give birth helped me stay calm and confident. I trusted her knowledge and experience. This birth happened fast, and Mary Ann's support made it more manageable. She was like a lighthouse in a storm, a steadying force and a guide. Mary Ann was not afraid, and her gentle touch was full of love. She never left my side; she whispered encouragement to me during the tough parts. She looked into my eyes, believing in me. I trusted her implicitly. After the birth, she checked on me, and we talked about my birth experience.

Mary Ann sometimes says she didn't do anything. I say it wasn't her doing; it was her being that helped. Her caring presence made everything better. Could I have done it without her? Yes, but it would have been harder.

Mary Ann has also helped me to be a better doula. The way she felt comfortable holding me has helped me hold others. The way she shared her thoughts in our birth story has helped me write nice stories for others. Having had the experience of someone just being with me through a difficult and painful experience helps me to understand that my quiet caring presence with others makes a difference to them.

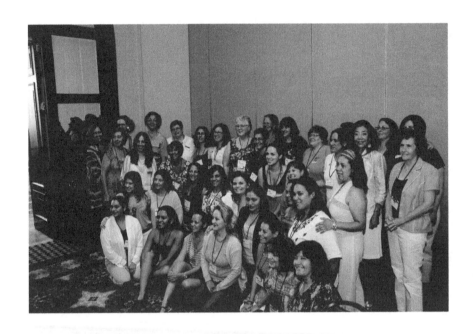

Photo 11. A gathering of doula trainers and childbirth educators at DONA International conference, Mexico, 2012.
Photo by Kyndal May.

Chapter Two

Becoming a Doula: Training and Early Practice[1]

> All primates find babies (the younger the better)
> fascinating, some more so than others.
>   Sarah Blaffer Hrdy[2]

Doulas often consider themselves unique among women because of their strong attraction to birth and caring for birthing women. In a training workshop, the instructor introduced an icebreaker exercise in which each doula trainee described what made her unique. Trainees mentioned such things as deep-sea diving, gourmet cooking, parachute jumping, or being the eldest of ten children. The trainer took her turn, and said:

> I love to be with women who are having babies. That's not unique here in this room, but in the world you'll find it is. What's unique is that we've been given this bug to be with women at this exceptional transition in their lives.[3]

---

1 This chapter is based on the author's sociological research on the history and experiences of doulas in the United States. The methodology is described in the Appendix.

2 Hrdy, S. B. (1999). *Mother nature: A history of mothers, infants and natural selection*. New York: Pantheon, p. 157.

3 For confidentiality reasons, doula trainers are not identified or described in detail.

This response unified the diverse attributes in the room and created a common bond among participants.

As this exercise, and my subsequent fieldwork showed, doulas understand themselves to be "special women" who have a deep interest and ability to care for other women during childbirth (Klaus, Kennell, & Klaus, 1993; Perez, 1990/1994). This interest and ability is often characterized as "uniquely female" in other parts of the training, but doula trainers readily acknowledge that not all women are interested in birth. Among the many factors that bring women to doula training are a long-standing interest in birth and an orientation toward caring for others.

Many women described their reaction to finding out about doulas and doula training as something they had always been looking for, but didn't know existed. They did not want or were unable to become a nurse, midwife, or physician, but they still wanted to be around births. When women heard about doulas, their response was often immediate. Doula Stacy Kinney shares her story.

> About four and a half years ago, I was getting ready for my office job one morning and there was a segment on *The Today Show* about doulas, and they were interviewing Marshall Klaus, and I was completely mesmerized. My husband came into the room and said, "Honey, you're going to be late for work," and I said, "It doesn't matter; I'm changing jobs." That was it; within a five-minute segment, I knew that I had found what I had been looking for all my life. I came home that night and said, "OK, get me on the Internet. I want to know everything I can find out about doulas." And by that night, I had already found a training and sent in my check.

Tiffany Smith said that after learning about doulas, she knew that this was "something I was destined to end up doing." She talks about a spiritual connection to birth, describing it as a "magnetic calling." Theresa Milton, who had read *Spiritual Midwifery*, a classic book published in 1977 on homebirth in her early teen years, recalls "When I saw the ad [for doula training], it was like a light went off in my head. I thought, 'I could do that.'"

Around the country, thousands of women have responded to advertisements for doula training. It takes much less time and money to become a certified doula than it does to become a certified childbirth educator. An unlicensed occupation, there are no formal requirements for calling oneself a doula. However, the steps to certification involve finding an organizationally approved training workshop locally (usually available within a day's drive of most metropolitan locations), paying between $400 to $700 for the course and materials, reading a few books, and spending a three to four days at a training (Gurevich, 2000). Attending the required number of births and filling in the paperwork to become certified takes a bit more time and effort. In many cities, local organizations provide guidance and support through the certification process. Motivated by the excitement generated at doula trainings, however, many new doulas find pregnant friends and relatives who are willing to have them attend their births in exchange for the certification requirements (and often take no fee for these births).

Women come to doula training out of an ideological commitment to caring for other women during birth, often shaped by their own experiences. Doula trainers say women come because some have had good birth experiences and want to share that with all women, and some have had bad experiences that they need to heal from. This divergence in birth experience and underlying motivation for attending the doula-training workshop can cause some tension. Sometimes, women become emotional as they share their stories. Trainers encourage personal reflection, reminding trainees to "think through why you're here. Those stories matter, there's a lot to be done in understanding your own story of what brought you here."

While instructors provide space for trainees to reflect on their own birth experiences, emotionally needy women may use excessive class time. More than one doula specifically noted that the main thing they did not like about the training was, as Alix Martin complained, "So many women wanted to talk about their own experiences."

Another doula training workshop observed in the course of my fieldwork took place in a school of midwifery where the course (or its equivalent) is a requirement for entering the midwifery program. The attendees ranged from an older married woman seeking to learn how to help at her daughter's upcoming hospital birth to a single 20-something with professional aspirations to become a midwife. Women bring a variety of personal and professional experience and knowledge to their doula practice. Doulas are also mothers, wives, yoga instructors, childbirth educators, homemakers, lactation consultants, massage therapists, nannies, nurses, midwives, photographers, postpartum doulas, childbirth educators, belly casters, writers, physician assistants, social workers, public health workers, teachers, psychologists, students, or retirees, among other occupations. These occupations are generally characterized by relatively low pay, a high degree of gender segregation (female dominated), and significant levels of emotional caregiving. In contrast, professions such as law or engineering are rarely represented among the trainees or doulas.

One notable exception is a woman who turned to doula practice after retirement from Microsoft. Peggy Foerch Fitzgerald of Seattle, Washington was featured in a *Wall Street Journal* Marketplace story about employees who move from high tech (and highly paid) to high passion (and highly altruistic) careers. The article describes how Fitzgerald transferred her corporate experience to her doula practice:

Ms. Fitzgerald learned to deal with teams of strong personalities while a Microsoft contract technical writer and fulltime program manager between 1989 and 1999. This talent comes in handy when she works with physicians on behalf of expectant mothers. Several of her clients have been Microsoft staffers who like her professionalism, empathy for their long hours, and ability to talk just like them. "The corporate world is a stepping stone," Ms. Fitzgerald observes. "Learn skills while you're there and go off and do something to give back. It's boring to just get, get, get" (Lublin, October 16, 2001).

Women who attend doula-training workshops span the age spectrum from the late teens to the mid-sixties and beyond. Most have had children; many plan to have them sometime in the future, and a small number are past childbearing age and have never had children. In some cities, liberal college environments provide a steady stream of young, single women majoring in women's studies, with aspirations to be midwives. In other locations, especially where women are recruited from the community via newspaper ads or notices in local libraries or churches, the trainees tend to be older, more mature, and with a variety of life and birth experiences.

Of the 44 women attending three doula trainings observed in my research, nearly 60% had children, 45% had attended at least one birth (other than their own) before taking the workshop, and 18% were engaged in other birth-related work as childbirth educators or lactation consultants. The differences between trainees at the two locations showed up clearly with the large number of aspiring midwives attending classes at the midwifery school. In contrast, the workshop taught by a former nurse attracted three nurses, while the classes taught in the midwifery school had none. In the three trainings observed, there were only three women of color. Among the 45 doulas interviewed in my study, just five identified as a racial/ethnic minority.

Those who attend a doula-training workshop are a self-selected group of mostly women who have a fascination with birth and a desire to support other women through the birth experience. Those who become certified and/or actively practice as doulas are an even more committed group. Overall, the typical practicing doula is female, white, married, with children.[4] She is likely to have a college degree or attended some college (Lantz, Low, Varkey, & Watson, 2005). She is largely self-educated in matters related to reproduction, and is a motivated learner and critical consumer. She is moderately to highly involved in organizations focusing on birth-related issues. She has limited direct experience with homebirth, but is passionate about how birth can be an empowering, positive experience for women. She may or may not be a self-declared feminist.

With regard to socioeconomic status, the doulas in my study fell within two major groups. A slight majority was lower-middle class, with working class origins. Eleven of the 45 doulas interviewed came from families where one or both parents had professional backgrounds and occupations. However, nearly all the doulas in the study indicated their mothers were full-time homemakers during their childhoods, even those whose mothers had professional training. These women resumed or attained professional work after the children were older.

In my analysis, I categorized doulas as belonging to one of three types: the career doula, the meaning seeker, and the committed newcomer. Sixteen women (35%) in this study were defined as career doulas. Generally older, they described themselves as the go-to support person within their familial and social networks. They were likely to say they were doulas "before they called it that." Many became interested in birth

---

4 Some doulas are male or transgender; however, the overwhelming majority of persons taking doula training identify as women. The recent focus on reproductive justice, anti-racism, and anti-oppression among birth workers is explored more fully in Monica Basile's dissertation (Basile, 2012). In this book, we use the gender terms most doulas we talked to were using at the time.

work through the experience of having their own children and by teaching childbirth education. Most, but not all of the career doulas in this group were also doula trainers. Many of these women had developed an entrepreneurial package of childbirth-related skills, goods, and services, such as massage, birth tub rentals, or photography, which provided ongoing access to a local childbirth community for referrals and networking. Some worked for birth-related businesses whose managers understood and accommodated irregular labor schedules and provided flexibility to their employee, the doula, with the on-call nature of the work. Career doulas have a long history of involvement in doula or birth-related organizational activities, often as founders of local or national associations.

The committed newcomers comprised just over half of the doulas in the study. The 24 doulas within this category came to doula practice after attending a doula-training workshop within the last five years. They were more likely to have recently had children, and as a result, practice less frequently than the career doulas. Committed newcomers were likely to move into other birth-related fields, such as childbirth education, as a result of their doula practice, rather than the reverse. In other ways, they shared the passion and commitment to this work with the career doulas, especially through their organizational involvement.

The final type, the "meaning seekers," was the least represented in the sample, and numbered four. This type was more representative of the trainee population which, for various reasons, decided not to continue into active doula practice or to become certified. These women, while having an uncertain future as doulas, were nevertheless ideologically driven by a passion for the ideal birth. They were also likely to express the most emotionally vulnerable feelings around birth. Some "meaning seekers" spoke of being adopted or feeling little connection to their mothers, as an example of their experiences. Doula trainers described the "meaning seekers" as women with little life experience or maturity; their motivations were highly emotional or ideological, and they were the group least likely to become certified and practice as a doula. "Meaning seekers" were more frequent among doulas with few to no organizational connections and were more often single and without children.

Given the relatively low cost and short time commitment required, attending doula training workshops is a realistic, manageable way for women to tangibly connect with a long-standing interest in birth. Many of the women interviewed in the study said they had been interested in birth and reproduction for as long as they could remember, and initially had aspirations to be doctors or midwives:

> When I was a little girl, I asked my mom who helped women have babies. She told me ob/gyn doctors. So I went around telling people I was going to be an ob/gyn (Selena Connor).

> About 20 years ago, my roommate had a couple of babies at home, and so I got to participate as a friend. I didn't know what I was doing, of course, but I enjoyed it, and after that experience I really wanted to become a midwife, and I looked into it, and the more I thought about having that ultimate responsibility for the life of the mother and child, the less appealing it seemed (Stacy Kinney).

> I've always been interested in birth, watching dairy goats give birth as a kid growing up on a farm (Tiffany Smith).

For various reasons, these women did not ultimately enter medical professions, whether obstetrics, midwifery, or veterinary science; however, they retained a long-held fascination with birth and upon hearing about doulas knew that this was a way they could be with women at births without the extensive time and costs of a clinical training program.

Trainers are more likely to have been providing labor support before such support was professionally organized; many were childbirth educators for some years prior to the emergence of widespread, organized doula training and practice. These women have described a sense of excitement and relief upon discovering newly forming doula organizations. "Wow, I'm not the only one," is a commonly remembered sentiment. It's interesting to note that providing labor support or playing an active role at births was not initially seen as a feature of childbirth educators' roles[5]. Many women had been alone in their communities as the person who was attending births. Incredulous friends and relatives often asked why anyone would want to attend women at births.

Finding others who were drawn to birth validated their passion. Most women who were doula trainers began by providing labor support for students in their childbirth education classes. They moved into teaching doula training workshops for the additional income, as well as for the external validation of the importance of their work. It also gave them a constantly replenished community of women to share experiences with and another outlet to express their passion for birth.

What Trainees Learn in Doula Training

Through an intense four-day workshop, doula trainers convey the definition of the doula role[6], present the medical and emotional consequentiality of doula-attended births, and in particular demonstrate how doulas accomplish their job of providing "physical, emotional and informational support to

5 This may have been one reason why ICEA, for example, did not want to sponsor labor support workshops in the late 1980s when Penny Simkin approached them with this request, as noted in Chapter One.

6 Here the doula role described comes from DONA International. Other doula organizations adopt similar definitions of the doula role.

the laboring woman while protecting the memory of her birth experience."

In a typical DONA doula training, participants learn how to provide labor support through a variety of educational modalities: by listening to lectures and stories, watching videos, engaging in role-play exercises focusing on communication skills or hands-on exercises to learn physical comfort measures, filling out questionnaires, and writing letters to each other. The participation is active, lively, and engaged. Women are there because they really want to be. The training is intentionally emotionally focused. Women cry, laugh, and bond with each other. The class roster is shared from the beginning to encourage future connections.

Doulas and the Historical, Intuitive Role of Women at Childbirth

Doula care is presented as a return to the community-based, woman-centered care that existed prior to the shift from home to hospital births in the early part of the century (Blue, 1994). In conveying this message, doula trainers employ a rhetoric that presumes a collectively shared, community-centered support of women's birthing experiences. This rhetoric asserts that birthing has been women's work—that women intuitively know how to birth, but our current culture has developed birth models centered around obstetric practices that interfere with intuitive and shared knowledge. Throughout the workshops, doula trainers present an alternative model for how woman-centered support can reclaim a place within medicalized childbirth in Western cultures.

One trainer introduces a film shown in many doula trainings, *The Timeless Way,* by saying:

Where have we come from? I have the belief, that if in most places, most people have an idea about what is true, it probably is. See what you can find of the consensus about birth and what we know to be true. What can we learn from our sisters?

The film describes archeological and anthropological research about birth practices and beliefs, including the ubiquity of woman-supported births and laboring in upright postures. After the historical review, the film concludes: "This age old wisdom is now available in American hospitals." Trainees are left with the message that supportive care in childbirth is what women have always done, and naturally know how to do.

Doula trainers use this universal and timeless approach to birth not only as a rationale for their current role at births, but as one way to connect with women from different cultural contexts than their own. In one doula training, the trainer quoted Henri Nouwen, a Catholic theologian who writes about the scaffolding of the self. She told the class that the scaffolding—our position, title, social graces, manners, clothing, furniture, and our neighborhood—comprises the social self. But, as she says, "In birth all this is stripped away—all that is her is laid bare." Positing an essential nature to birthing women is a typical strategy in doula trainings.

Other trainers employ a schematic illustrating the universality of emotional needs in labor using Maslow's hierarchy of need developed as a teaching tool by Penny Simkin. Women, described in training lectures, are collapsed into "mom" or the "generic woman." Very few cross-cultural examples are used except to highlight the superiority of the "natural" way, the way of women in cultures where medical resources have been or are currently scarce. The relatively higher morbidity and mortality of these women and infants is not highlighted, however. Furthermore, the contradictions embedded in this essential view of culture—that birth never changes and women's bodies naturally know how to birth—are never made explicit.

When the diversity of women's perspective is acknowledged, doula trainers imply some views are a byproduct of misinformation. For example, one doula trainer described how the success of 19th century campaigns for pain relief in childbirth had unintended consequences: "The suffragettes marched in the streets for the right to have pain relief in labor. They didn't know what the trade-offs would be." Had the suffragettes understood how women would be treated while under Twilight Sleep (an amnesiac mixture of scopolamine and morphine), or its physically damaging effects on women or infants, they would not have fought for it, and would have instead advocated for bringing their female friends with them for labor support.

Selena Connor, a young-looking, African-American woman who was often mistaken for a friend rather than a doula tells a story about her experience helping a young Vietnamese client during her labor in a local hospital. The woman spoke no English, and Selena spoke no Vietnamese. Her client was in active labor, feeling very physically uncomfortable, expressing this with occasional loud outbursts of pain and fear. Selena said she spoke softly encouraging words, looked deeply in her client's eyes, stroked her hands, and the woman's discomfort lessened to the obvious relief of the medical staff present. Selena could tell her client did not understand what the obstetric clinicians were saying about her progress and the possible interventions under consideration. For some reason, there was no interpreter, even though all non-English speaking patients have a right to an interpreter in U.S. hospitals. Selena recalls:

A doctor entered, observed for a few minutes, and then asked me to tell her, in fairly complex terms, what he proposed to do. I informed him I could not do that, because I did not speak Vietnamese. He looked shocked, and said that he couldn't believe I could get "that woman calmed down without speaking her language."

Doulas love to hear stories like this, as they assert the doula's universal connection with women in labor, the idea that birth transcends language, and that women can connect with other women on this birth plane alone, regardless of significant differences between them, in this case language.

What Doulas Do Not Learn

Early debates among doula pioneers involved whether to incorporate clinical skills in the labor support role. Some felt strongly that if the doula could assess cervical dilation, laboring women would be able to stay at home longer before going to the hospital. Others felt that claiming such skills incurred responsibility and liability that was unnecessary for the overall functioning and success of the labor support role. From its inception, DONA International adopted the position that while trainees/doulas may have past training from previous careers or future aspirations to be a medical professional, the DONA International doula "… does not perform clinical or medical tasks, such as taking blood pressure or temperature, fetal heart tone checks, vaginal examinations or postpartum clinical care" (DONA International Standards of Practice, 2000).[7]

Within this strong organizational framework, the medical aspects of the doula role were not debated much in doula training workshops. However, trainees learned that what "counts" as medical information may not be immediately obvious. A doula trainer instructs her class: "Do not interpret

---

7 Current documents are available from http://www.dona.org/aboutus/standards_birth.php.

for her what she's seeing on the fetal monitor. Say, "Let's ask the nurse next time she comes in." You can help mom get the answer she needs, but not from you."

Even when the doula has been to many births and feels she has some ability to interpret the fetal monitor, she is supposed to defer to the authority of the obstetric clinicians. Although in practice doulas negotiate with obstetric clinicians in ways that blur this seemingly strict boundary, in the training, the lines are drawn very clearly. Warning stories from trainers illustrate the danger of providing medical advice.

You could seriously endanger her health if you suggest things to start her labor. You can point out things in a book, but you should also say, "Before you try any of these, check with your care provider just to be sure there is nothing to contraindicate the use of this."

Trainees learn that their non-medical role is what distinguishes them from maternity care providers, and this fills a gap within the current hospital provision of childbirth support. Closing this gap takes two forms: first, the doula's focus is specifically on the laboring woman's emotional and physical comfort needs, rather than clinical issues. Second, the doula provides continuous presence and personalized attention to one woman, in contrast to the competing demands of the clinicians present, whether nurse, midwife, or physician.

In most hospitals, obstetric nurses are assigned more than one patient, but even in hospitals with mandated one-to-one nursing care for women in active labor or receiving certain medications, women with long labors receive care from a number of different nurses with shift changes, dinner breaks, or emergencies interfering with nursing continuity of care. As this aspect of the doula's role was elaborated during a training, one trainee remarks, "This medical approach makes me angry." The doula trainer responds:

It's important to realize that we [as doulas] can evaluate births in a different way. I find the nurses take the power away from the mom. As a doula, you take the time, without the nurse around. I don't find the doctor taking power away, it's the nurses, and they go away. I find the power comes from the consistent person.

Trainees learn that in American hospitals, amid high rates of medical intervention in even normal births, the emotional needs of women are often secondary to the monitoring technology and documenting requirements, which demand nursing attention. They learn that doulas are uniquely positioned to meet women's emotional needs during the labor and birth experience. They also learn, as the above exchange illustrates, that they are simultaneously powerful and powerless in the hospitalized birth setting.

Birth as Normal and the Midwifery Model of Care

In addition to the focus on the non-medical aspects of their own role, doulas learn that pregnancy and childbirth are normal, non-pathological life events. This notion is embedded in the midwifery model of care, which is conveyed very strongly in most doula training workshops. In the first two days of training, which are required for those with no prior work experience as a nurse or childbirth educator, trainees are informed about the midwifery model and learn the basics of childbirth physiology. The midwifery model of care can be described as a holistic approach that attends to the diverse aspects of pregnancy and birth: physical, emotional, spiritual, social, economic, cultural, and sexual. All these elements are briefly introduced in doula training with the emphasis on birth as a natural physiological process occurring in healthy women, with fewer medical interventions yielding better outcomes for both women and their babies.

The full elaboration of birth as a non-medical event can be a new concept for some trainees who have come to birth through their experiences helping family members or friends and who have had medically managed experiences in hospitals. Such an approach to pregnancy and birth comes as a paradigm shift. Tiffany Smith, a nurse when she attended the doula-training workshop, recalls how this affected her orientation toward hospital births:

Medical management is part and parcel of what I do as a nurse. Going in as a nurse, medications seemed natural. In my evolution through douladom, I learned how profoundly medications affect labor. I did not expect to learn this. I went to two out-of-hospital births and came home elated. From the hospital births, I would always come home feeling frustrated.

Despite the emphasis on their non-medical role, doulas are nevertheless expected to be conversant with standard medical practices surrounding birth.[8] Trainees learn about pain medications used in labor and the kinds of information they are expected to give their clients prenatally and during labor to help them make informed decisions. Although critical of the unnecessary use of medical interventions, trainees are expected to be familiar with their indications. Knowledge of anatomy and physiology of childbirth is encouraged in order to understand how to help labor progress in situations where the baby is not in an optimal position. Some women with little birth experience or knowledge before the course find the amount of information overwhelming, lamenting that it is too much material to absorb in so short a time.

---

8 In Rebecca Klassen's study on women choosing homebirth, she found that women were very comfortable and knowledgeable with medical terminology. She attributed this to the hegemony of biomedicine (Klassen, 2001).

Doula trainers in this study relied on two major sources to convey to trainees the medical and emotional consequentiality of labor support, and these remain central texts in the DONA International approved reading list. The first is a required reading, *Mothering the Mother: How a Doula can Help You Have a Shorter, Easier, and Healthier Birth*[9], by DONA International founders and researchers Marshall Klaus, John Kennell, and Phyllis Klaus that distills the findings of clinical research trials on doula-attended births.

These and subsequent studies found that not only was mother-infant bonding positively affected, but in addition: "the presence of a doula reduces the overall caesarean rate by 50 percent, length of labor by 25 percent, oxytocin use by 40 percent, pain medication by 30 percent, the need for forceps by 40 percent, and requests for epidurals by 60 percent" (Klaus, Kennell & Klauss, 1993, p. 51).

Trainers emphasize one important finding of the early clinical trials: that women in the control group, with a female research assistant observing and taking notes but not providing active labor support also experienced significant differences in length of labor, cesarean rates, and epidural use compared to the treatment group.

The other primary source used by doula trainers to highlight the emotional consequentiality of birth is the research study by childbirth educator, author, and another founder of Doulas of North America/DONA International, Penny Simkin (1991, 1992a), described in Chapter One. Trainers spend a great deal of time discussing the emotional aspects of birth. Simkin's research findings emphasize that

---

9 Reissued in 2002 with a new title: *The Doula Book: How a Trained Labor Companion Can Help You Have a Shorter, Easier, and Healthier Birth.*

a woman's satisfaction with the memory of her birth is influenced more by how she was treated than by the number or type of medical interventions she experienced. Feminist social scientists Bonnie Fox and Diana Worts also arrive at this conclusion in their research interviews conducted with women four days to two weeks after giving birth. They found that "social support not only enabled women to deal with the pain and anxiety of their first labors and deliveries, [but] even substituted for medical assistance" (Fox & Worts, 1999, p. 341). Their research also claims that women's feelings about their births were not strongly correlated with interventions or physical complications from the birth itself, but rather with the level of social support they received during and after the birth, including the presence of a generally supportive partner.

The unique contribution of Simkin's research is the documentation of women's long-term memories of their birth experience. She contacted women from her childbirth classes who had given birth to their first child between 1968 and 1974, and asked them to fill out a questionnaire and write their birth story. Simkin then compared these questionnaires and stories with the ones the women had given her 15 to 20 years prior. She also conducted interviews during which the memories were discussed and discrepancies were elaborated upon. As she compared the data from the two time periods, Simkin found that women's memories were "vivid and deeply felt," and that exact details of comments, smells, and colors were retained. After analysis, Simkin divided the 20 women into two groups based on their current satisfaction with their births. She reports the factors associated with satisfaction:

> … have more to do with the way they conduct themselves, and the way they are treated, than with the actual clinical features of their labor. Short and long labors, and use and non-use of interventions, were represented in both groups.

The women with positive feelings today recall being well cared for and supported by the doctor and nurse, whereas those with negative feelings today tend to recall negative interactions with staff (Simkin, 1991, p. 209).

The central message that doula trainers convey to trainees comes from the results of the research described above, particularly Simkin's. This message claims that supportive, emotional care has been found to positively impact medical outcomes and long-term satisfaction of birthing women. Trainers provide dramatic and graphic descriptions as they relate these research findings, emphasizing what women do and do not remember about their births, as this doula trainer does:

She'll have vivid snapshot memories of the birth. She won't remember exactly the graph of labor. She'll have snapshot memories of key moments where her soul is laid bare, and she's naked, vulnerable, and ready to be inculcated with messages to her psyche, her inner core, about her values. She'll remember 50 years later the kindness and the cruelty shown to her.

The emotional and physical vulnerability of the woman during birth is emphasized, as is the opportunity for someone to fill the gaps left between the "snapshot memories." How does a doula protect and nurture that birth memory? One answer is embedded within the mother-infant bonding research. The medical researchers' insights into how to accomplish supportive care in labor are elevated in this story told by a doula trainer:

Marshall Klaus came to Seattle and a doula wanted to know "What can we do to encourage bonding?" His answer was: "Be very kind to the mother." That's something all of us can do. We can't remember or know the right thing to say or do but we can always do that one thing. We can always be kind.

This simultaneously raised expectation of birth outcomes, both medically and emotionally, with the seemingly effortless means to accomplish it can leave new doulas feeling either comfortable and reassured, or fearful of saying or doing the wrong thing.

This concern is reinforced when doula trainers caution that the emotional power and consequentiality of birth can be traumatic as well as euphoric: "We think of peak as a high point, but it has as much potential to be a low point." The trainer related that women in Simkin's study who comprised the high-satisfaction group described birth in terms of accomplishment. She told the class that the birth either affirmed or changed the woman's self-concept. Doula trainers carefully weave their lessons to demonstrate the power of a positive birth without putting the entire onus for achieving this on the doula. One trainer draws an emotional lesson from these research results, asking "How can anyone walk out of a place after having a baby and NOT feel a sense of achievement?" The trainer answers her own question.

She had a baby, she brought forth new life, she sacrificed herself and something they did or said made the woman walk out without a sense of accomplishment. That's a crime, that's a shame. That's something we can do as doulas, I don't care even if it's born at 20 weeks, it's a precious thing to see created in your body—the cells knit together. Penny's study reaffirmed my work, it's not just another day. (The woman next to me is sniffling, and as another class member gets up to get a drink, she puts her hand on the crying woman's shoulder). Doulas help protect the memory of the birth. How will she remember this in her first retelling when she calls her mother?

A trainee responds to this story with a question about what she might have said to a client who had called her mother immediately after the birth, full of elation. The client's mother had no positive words for her, and as a result, the new mother became deflated, losing her sense of accomplishment. The doula trainer replies, "If a woman doesn't have that kind of mother, the doula is that mothering presence. How might we think about helping her to insulate herself from that person?"

The trainee acknowledges, "I didn't see that coming ahead of time." The trainer asks if she had read *Mothering the Mother*:

Did you see the clinical trials? Were you surprised? In talking about the control group in the Houston study, the laboring women talked about the woman behind the curtain (the woman taking notes) as "my guardian angel." You're going to be better than the woman behind the curtain. I promise you that. Even if you hold her hand and say, "You're doing good" once an hour, you're going to affect clinical outcomes and make that woman's birth experience better.

By conflating the trained doula with the "woman behind the curtain," the trainer affirms the power of the doula just by being perceived as a caring person. She also makes an assertion that the doula's words and actions during a time-limited period—birth and postpartum—can fundamentally affect a woman's self-perception with more significance than her own mother. The doula trainer continues:

The untrained labor support person holding a woman's hand made a huge difference. If we go to the hospital and say we have this new technology, it would do xyz, and it only costs $400 for this technology, who wouldn't snap that up? Some of you love the medical part of birth and go on to be midwives. This is my love, this emotional support is important work and that's been shown, so has midwifery, to have incredible results for women.

She does not offer information about the conditions under which the women in the early trials labored. One review of these early trials notes:

> The women in the Texas study received appalling treatment by the standard of any industrialized country ... they labored in 12-bed wards that "had insufficient privacy to allow visitors ... patients were usually in the presence of strangers ... and were attended by professional staff who could not speak their language (Richards, 1992, p. 40).

The value of supportive care in such a situation is likely to improve outcomes by virtue of its relative absence in the standard-care groups.

What does it mean for emotional support to be compared to a "new technology" that costs a mere $400 and has been shown to have "incredible results" for women? Doula trainers work hard to convey the emotional rewards to trainees, but struggle to work this compensation into a rational economic framework that typically devalues the human element of care, often in hospital settings where birth is oriented to as a routine event. Thus trainers rely heavily on stories, videos, and personal accounts from guest speakers—women who recently had a baby with a doula—to convey the emotional power of supportive care to trainees.

For the most part, doula trainers provide references to research studies to support their claims that non-interventive births are optimal and that labor support has positive outcomes. Where the research claims end and the value statements begin is more complex. Underlying the training workshop is a strong belief in birth as a vulnerable time, when women are "stripped bare" and emotionally exposed to others. A universality of vulnerability is presumed in the physical act of labor. Nuance, cultural, and individual variation tend to be subsumed within this overarching belief.

In instances such as the one above involving a non-affirming mother, empirical questions as to whether the doula's affirmation of the birthing woman's effort will override her own mother's dismissal of it are left unexamined. In several analyses of birth stories, scholars critically elaborate the mediated contours of memory—these stories are not static, but are altered through prior and subsequent experience, as well as the specific cultural and social contexts of a birth experience (Adams, 1994; Cosslett, 1994; Klassen, 2001; Pollock, 1999). Doula analyses of birth stories, however, focus on their continuity over time, independent of the social or interactional context of their telling (Simkin, 1991, 1992a).

Other dilemmas within the doula role emerge and become potentially problematic in two significant ways. First, as mentioned earlier, the strong emphasis placed on long-term emotional consequentiality of how women were treated at the birth raises concerns among new doulas. Trainers address these concerns through examples of caring that rely on women's natural intuitive knowledge on how to care and by asserting that "just being there" makes a difference.

Second, the emphasis on clinical trial results, in conditions very different from those in which most trainees will work as doulas, raises the statistical point known as the ecological fallacy: applying aggregate results to individual cases. However, the ecological fallacy, the structural context of most U.S. births, and limits to the doula's efficacy are not typically discussed in doula training workshops. As a result, many women finish the training believing the births they will attend will produce similar outcomes to those promised from the clinical trials and when this does not happen, over time, many become disheartened and frustrated with the real limitations of the doula role.

Doula Values and Dilemmas: Unconditional Support and the Role of Advocacy

Doula trainers present the view that labor support should include unconditional emotional acceptance of women and their choices, practical physical assistance, and as much information as women need to make decisions that are best for them. Although trainers stress that birth is "not just another day" in a woman's life and provide scientific rationale for asserting the medical and emotional consequentiality of continuous labor support, they also emphasize the importance of not judging women's choices for their births or advocating one's own beliefs on behalf of other women in medical settings.

Despite underscoring the importance of respecting the birthing woman's choice of care provider, birth location, and any desire or plan for pain medications, doula training workshops set up a contradiction faced by many trainees who have just learned about a model of birth that posits midwifery, out-of-hospital birth, and low interventions as optimal. Thus, communicating how to hold strong beliefs and yet not advocate for them is not always a simple matter, even if the trainer is clear about it, as Penny Simkin describes.

It's a tricky one. I mean, I feel very clear on it, I feel very clear on it. Personally, I think getting it across in the trainings is difficult. A lot of people are drawn to birth as birth advocates. They love natural birth, and midwife-attended birth, or they are baby advocates ... where they really want to make sure that the baby gets the best possible start, as they see it. So I think they have a stake and a cause that they try to promote, and it's very hard not to advocate for that cause (P. Simkin, personal communication, February 15, 2000).

Doula trainers clearly stress that while advocacy is an important part of the doula role, it does not mean starting a confrontation with obstetric clinicians at the woman's hospital birth. As one trainer puts it:

… there are two avenues for our advocacy. One is what we do professionally as doulas. We can advocate for change on behalf of maternity care procedures—when NOT attending women in labor. Two is what we do when attending women in labor. A doula in the labor room is worth three doulas in the waiting room. Ask questions and model good communication. Help mom get the kind of birth she wants, not the kind you think she should want. Remind her and encourage her to speak up on her own behalf. Be careful not to speak for her.

Doula trainers rely heavily on stories to get this point about advocacy across. Often the story comes from their own experiences and highlights their own mistakes. A doula trainer reveals, somewhat sheepishly:

I did it the wrong way once. As the doctor picked up the scissors, I said, "Oh no, she doesn't want an episiotomy," and the mom said, "Oh, I don't care, get this baby out." I felt stupid, and he [the doctor] thought I was a meddling idiot.

Despite the clarity with which the doula trainers present the issue, it can be difficult to follow this advice in the highly charged, emotional setting of a medicalized birth[10]. Trainers stress that the doula's emotional reaction to what is happening, especially anger, should not lead her to act inappropriately in

---

10 None of the doulas in this study complained about midwife-attended births in the same way.

the setting—whether she sees obstetric clinicians acting in a disrespectful manner or giving what the doula considers to be misleading or inaccurate information about a proposed intervention. Inappropriate actions by doulas in these contexts, according to the DONA model, would include confronting obstetric clinicians about their disrespectful words or actions, or contradicting their information, either in their presence or when they leave the room.

This leads to the question among new doulas about their role in ensuring or assisting their client in informed decision-making or informed consent, especially in the frequent situations where clinical providers do not provide information about the risks or benefits of a given procedure at the time that an intervention is about to occur. Trainees learn, however, that informed consent is not the responsibility of the doula, but of the maternity care provider. Yet depending on a clinician's particular practice style or immediate understanding of the situation, a physician or nurse may not take the time to inform the woman about what is happening.

In the following example, a doula trainer describes how to be an effective advocate in the case of newborn complications. In her scenario, immediately after birth, the baby has been taken, screaming, to the corner of the room to be attended by clinicians, none of whom give the woman or her partner an explanation. In her story, the trainer implies she knows what the mom is feeling, but not verbalizing, while this is happening.

This mom is saying, "What about my moment?" Well, the doula can say, "This baby wants his mama." Can you say that? We have to say it good naturedly, and can't really say it if baby's not okay. Think about how you might do that.

The class brainstorms other approaches to this, and similar scenarios.

There are two dimensions to the doula's informational role, both of which are problematic for doula practice. One is whether the doula can claim to have information that is considered specialized medical knowledge, as the trainer notes in the case above—if the baby's not okay, you can't encourage the woman to ask for her baby, and thus imply the clinician's actions are unwarranted. The second dimension is the underlying assumption that with "unbiased and accurate" information, the woman will make choices about her birth that the doula would likely agree with. Doula trainers take special pains to disabuse doulas of this second. Trainers stress that women who decide to have an intervention or pain medication or to formula-feed have good reasons, and doulas should not second-guess them.

Trainers emphasize the distinction between how doulas talk about women's desires and values in the prenatal visit when they have time to question the woman and offer more information to aid her decision-making, and how to manage this dilemma in the interactional moment regarding a procedure that is disagreeable to either the woman or the doula. Penny Simkin elaborates the latter dilemma:

See that's what a lot of new doulas think, "If I shut up here, I'm letting my client down; letting them get away with murder," all that stuff. But it's by picking your battles, and remembering whose birth this is—if the mother doesn't choose to speak up, then maybe there's another value that is driving her, it might be fear of the doctor, who knows, but she may rather not have a confrontation. If she doesn't want that, then she's not choosing to enter that fray. I could be doing more harm than good. There are times when I've just had to hold on to a woman through something that she didn't want, [but isn't objecting to at the time], and I feel like I'm abetting, but at least better than abetting, giving her some nurturing and love through something awful, or I risk getting kicked out, and leaving her totally alone. You know it's, ichh...[INT: It puts the doula in a very difficult spot...] It's a very difficult spot, and we have to swallow hard, and that's one reason we have our groups, so that she [the doula] has someplace to go with all this rage that can be generated in situations like that (P. Simkin, personal communication, February 15, 2000).

The rage that is generated can be quite intense. Doulas turn to support groups, both in person and online, to express their feelings of anger and frustration. Although in the abstract the doula's advocacy and informational roles seem clear, the interactional accomplishment of this role in particularly stressful decision points is complex and is further discussed in Chapter Four.

What Kind of Advocate are You?

Doulas' reasons for doing this work, and what it means to them, center on the significance of three interconnected aspects: a woman's experience of birth, the birth itself, and the baby that emerges. Doulas vary in the degree to which they hold any of these aspects in greater priority; one way that doulas attempt to judge this for themselves has been through a self-assessment developed by Penny Simkin, used in some but not all doula training workshops.[11]

Several doulas have referred to Simkin's typology when responding to questions about why they do this work. The self-assessment asks "What kind of advocate are you? Baby? Birth? Woman?" and begins:

---

11 Materials and curricular content may vary across training workshops because doula trainers submit individualized training curricula for DONA International approval. Other doula training organizations may use different curricula, and may not rely as heavily on Simkin's material as do DONA trainers.

My main reason for being active in childbirth-related work is:

   a. The baby. I want to be sure the baby's entrance into the world is as safe and caring as possible.
   b. Natural childbirth. I want to be sure that safe, midwife-attended, low-intervention, out-of-hospital birth choices are always available to women.
   c. The woman. I want to be sure that women have choices and the freedom to make those choices, even if they are not ones I would make.

The assessment then includes five more items, each of which begins with the statement: "I feel comfortable working with women who ..." Doulas are instructed to place a 0 if they do not feel comfortable at all with this statement; a checkmark if they are okay with it; and a double checkmark if they prefer to work with a woman who has the attitude or engages in the behavior under consideration.

These statements include attitudes and behaviors for which pregnant women may be morally evaluated by others, such as planning an epidural, being afraid of hospitals, planning to circumcise their sons (or daughters), smoking cigarettes, using marijuana, believing that immunizations do more harm than good, placing their baby in daycare, or worrying that the baby may interfere with other priorities in life. The self-assessment says there is no right or wrong, but that:

> The answers may help you recognize whether you have strong preferences (biases?) that will keep you from providing excellent care for all clients. If so, you should restrict your care to those with whom you are comfortable. Think about it (Simkin, 1997).

The baby advocate is someone who agrees with (a) and who also prefers to work with someone who believes that many or all hospital routines are dangerous to their babies or unnecessary; that immunizations do more harm than good; and that infant formula and antibiotics have toxic effects. These advocates have the most 0s in items where women engage in behaviors, such as alcohol consumption, smoking, formula feeding, or are in abusive relationships; or in items where the woman does not want her baby to room in during the hospital stay, wants to return to work after the baby is born, and plans to put the baby in daycare.

The birth advocate is someone who agrees with (b), where the checked items include preferences working with women who are afraid of the hospital and/or obstetricians; plan a home or birth-center birth; prefer midwives; fear epidurals and episiotomies; will read, attend classes, and make a birth plan; desire a natural childbirth, and see labor and birth as a personal challenge, a chance to prove themselves. These advocates have more 0s in items where the woman plans an early epidural or wants an elective cesarean; may not attend childbirth classes; and doesn't really care how they give birth, as long as they and the baby are okay.

The woman advocate is someone who agrees with (c) and has many checks and double checks in all categories and few zeros. When doulas in my study mentioned this self-assessment, they predominantly placed themselves within the woman advocate category. Even when they identified as a baby advocate or stated a preference for unmedicated birth, doulas nevertheless highlighted the centrality of the birthing woman's right to make decisions with as much information about potential risks and benefits of proposed interventions as possible. No doula in my study indicated she had any convictions so great as to not be able to accept someone else's decisions as right for them. Rae Messenger is typical of many doulas in her response to a question about her view of birth:

> When we took that test, Penny's quiz, birth advocate, women's advocate, baby advocate, I'm a "birth advocate." You take these multiple-choice questions, and then according

to how many you have in a certain category, that leads you to a certain way. When I see women who say, "I'm going to get the epidural as soon as I can," that doesn't bother me. I don't have a campaign about anything, unless it would be that the mother has an opportunity to know what kind of impact those procedures might have. And when I do my prenatal visit, I always tell her it's her decision—not what I want, not what the doctor or nurse tells her to do. I want to provide that little space where she can know she decided ... I want that experience to be open for her to experience it, not based on what she decided at some time before she really knew what the facts really were going to be about. So that's how I see more of the birth advocate, the woman may go through it naturally, I like to encourage that, but I also feel if they get to a point where they can't do it, I don't want them to feel that, "My god, now I failed, I can't do anything."

Rae later notes that she may have the categories mixed up, which, in fact, she does. Her description of her advocacy matches the assessment's definition of the woman advocate, which she incorrectly remembered as "more militant against interventions ... with a woman's advocate, you decide what you're going to do, and by God, no one's going to make you do anything else." Rae, however, remembers the baby advocate fairly accurately: "The baby advocate, for instance, is about interventions, no vitamin K shot." She goes on to say that these two views are much too "confrontive (sic), it's not a comforting, natural kind of thing. If they want to feel that way, as a birth advocate, I want to allow them that expression, but also a chance to change their mind about what they decided."

The majority of doulas in my study claimed to be woman advocates, although some, like Rae, were unclear about the distinction between the categories. The underlying focus of their doula work was the woman. Maisy Simmons is emphatic about her position:

We did this little test, you know, are you a woman advocate, baby advocate, or a birth advocate, and I'm a woman advocate. I'm all about her and what she wants. I love the babies, and birth can be gorgeous and wonderful, but I want her to feel good about her body afterwards.

Even those doulas who were strong baby advocates found it difficult to separate this position from being a woman advocate as well, as Lorie Nelson shares:

A lot of people think about birth about the baby, and I do, and I think about the transformation of the mother, you know, of a woman into the mother. And what a powerful, powerful time that is. And I remember my sister in law—who is a childbirth educator, and who has subsequently become a doula—at one time she said to me, "Lorie, in the birthing community there are baby advocates and then there are mother advocates." This is not verbatim, but it was something like that, there are people on this side, and people on that side, and I think she was sort of coming from like the baby advocate idea. I must say that where I'm at in the present moment, is that to be a baby advocate, I have to be a mother advocate. Because that mother is that baby's God for the moment, you know, until this soul can cognate and differentiate and individuate, and one day recognize that their parents were not God, and that they could have their own relationship with God, these parents are this baby's God who will nourish, protect, guide, feed, you know, so to me, the impact I can make with the family, particularly the mother, is very important.

Unlike the biomedical conception of a maternal/fetal split, with two patients—two competing sets of interests, rights and needs—the doula conceptualization, as articulated by Lorie, struggles to keep these entities interconnected in recognition of their ongoing relationship after birth until the eventual separation and individuation of the child. This view is supported by a strong assumption that the care women receive at birth will in turn affect how they feel about and care for their babies. This view of "mothering the mother" is highly promoted at doula training workshops. The message from Klaus and Kennell's mother-infant bonding research emerges most strongly here, when the notion of "being kind to the mother" means that the (woman) mother will, in turn, exhibit more attachment to the baby.

These three types of advocacy represent rigid points along a fairly fluid yet relatively consistent spectrum of beliefs and practices about not only which battles to fight in the labor room, or how to assess one's own beliefs and boundaries regarding the kind of women one might accept as clients, but also about their view of women as mothers. Lorie Nelson, like many other doulas, omitted any mention of the term "woman," and used "mother." To be a baby advocate, she must be a mother advocate.

While most doulas expressed a personal preference for unmedicated, low-intervention childbirth, they were also quite adamant that they could support women's choices—the mothers' choices—as best for them. Roberta King is active in anti-abortion organizations, so baby advocacy drives, but does not determine, her stance toward the mother's decisions. Roberta explains her position.

I don't have an opinion. Basically, that's up to the mother. It's her decision. My training helps me help people make their own decisions. My personal choice would be little or no medication, simply for the baby's sake. I've been at a birth where had the mother chose medication, the baby would have had brain damage simply because the cord was wrapped around the neck, resulting in a lack of oxygen. Now because baby did not have medication, it was no problem. Therefore, the doctor said because the baby was not groggy, they did not have to do extraordinary measures to bring that baby back. If I am an advocate, it would be to help them to get through it without medication, but if they choose medication, I'm still there. I don't say, "Don't do that," but I do let them know that with medication there are dangers, real dangers for the baby, you know. And I still try to work with them, when they give them the epidural and lay them on their back. That doesn't help them. Then they tell them, "Well, you're not progressing." [INT: So do you feel differently about a birth where you've been able to help a woman have a baby without medication?] No. [INT: The emotional thing you get out of it is not different?] No, I feel emotionally satisfied if she had the birth that she needs.

In this way, doula accounts of what they do consistently reflect the DONA injunction to unconditionally support birthing women's choices. While the accounts are consistent, it is nevertheless in practice where the client will perceive the authenticity of the doula's unconditional support. At present there is no research examining how doula clients perceive their doula's support for choices that the doula considers ill-advised—or wrong.

Learning to Reframe the Birth Experience

Doulas learn in training that one of the most powerful ways they interact with their clients at births is by reframing what is happening from something that is negative or scary into something that highlights the normalcy of labor or the agency of the birthing woman. Trainers communicate the value of reframing events in order for the woman to have a story to tell that places her agency and her decisions at the center. Trainers acknowledge doulas are often present when the first telling of the birth story is announced to family members, especially when it occurs within minutes of the birth, via telephone, social media, email, or text. The injunction to "protect and nurture the birth memory" is conveyed at the training through a variety of means, not the least of which is hands-on physical comfort measures. What the doula says is as significant as what the doula does in shaping the tell-able story of that birth for the woman, her partner, and their families. Trainees learn that reframing can occur during birth itself when the woman experiences painful contractions or their unpleasant side effects. As one doula trainer shared, "We get happy as doulas about things she might not be happy about. Hard, long contractions, we're just so thrilled. When she vomits, we're like 'Yeah!'"

Negative experiences in everyday life—vomiting—are reframed into positive events in labor. Vomiting has a productive purpose: the spasms work to move the baby down and open up the cervix. Another reframing occurs when women feel embarrassed or inhibited about the possibility of defecating while pushing. One doula trainer offers, "When they're pushing their baby out, I give them permission. I say it's the 3 Ps of pushing: When you push and you poop, that's perfect."

In addition to reframing unpleasant physical side effects of labor, such as vomiting and defecating, doula trainers suggest emotionally reframing labor pain from something that is feared and avoidable to something that is normal and integral to the birth process. When the woman resists this reframing, trainers suggest doulas explore this further, and work from the emotional meaning the woman is giving to her labor experience, as in this example from a workshop exchange:

Ask the woman, "What was going through your mind during that contraction?" Asking, "Anything else?" is a good way to get more. Sometimes her analogy is yucky.

When I asked, "What was going through your mind during that contraction?" one woman answered, "It felt like a big black slithery creature going over my tummy with a sharp tail." Can anybody reframe this? [A trainee quips: "Call Orkin,[12]" provoking laughter]. The doula trainer continued, "How about, 'I think we can drown it in the tub. Would you like to move to the bath?"

Trainers acknowledge that labor and the effort involved in reframing it is hard work for the doula and the laboring woman. When women get stuck in an unproductive place, trainees are encouraged to suggest the woman do something different from what she is currently doing. "If their eyes are closed, have them open their eyes, and tell them to look at their belly." The trainer provides an example of a mantra to visualize the uterus not as the object of pain and fear, but something wondrous. As she begins the visualization, her voice turns soft and melodious, gentle but confident: "Say, 'look at that big beautiful pink skin, it's my uterus, it's my uterus, time to shine, it's shining, just blow.'" She instructs the trainees to always try and reframe, but concedes that sometimes they will feel at a loss. In such instances, trainers reassure, a tried-and-true reframing technique is to "get her back to reality. It's not foreign or scary, just your baby coming out."

In addition to explicit reframing techniques, trainees learn the power and the limits of their observations to help them make sense of the woman's experience. A doula trainer explains what they may see:

Observe how she breathes and talks through contractions. Watch her behavior—does she pause, is her faced scrunched up or in a beautiful trance? How is she breathing, what sort of facial expression or sounds is she making? Some women are quiet and still; others vocalize a lot.

---

12 Making reference to a pest-control business.

Trainees are told observation can be a tool, but only when it is done without assumptions about where a woman is or what she is feeling in labor. A doula trainer ruefully related a self-deprecating story about one client who didn't say a thing during labor but afterwards, "She told me my voice was like fingernails on a chalkboard." The trainer learned from this that observations alone do not necessarily indicate what is going on in the laboring woman's mind or heart.

Another example trainers relate is that when a laboring woman moans loudly, it doesn't necessarily mean she's not coping. It is important for the doula to ask the woman how she feels. A doula trainer says, "If we ask her, she may say, 'It feels good to make my voice go like that." Then it's the doula's job to make everyone around her feel okay with her vocalizations.'"

Reframing women's emotional experiences through verbal affirmations is essential. This is accomplished by acknowledging the woman's pain.

> You can say things like: "I know this is painful. This is hard work." Praise the woman's effort: "You're doing wonderfully. You are so strong." Validate her decisions, provide an informational context that can be especially useful when the woman's wishes for her birth cannot be fully realized: "You've been laboring for so long, it's been 36 hours of painful back labor. With an epidural you can rest and let your cervix finish dilating. You are making the right decision for yourself."

In certain situations, as in the case of sexual abuse survivors, trainers stress the importance for doulas to be conscious of the words and images they use during reframing. In the past ten years, the issue of how sexual abuse survivors experience birth has become a central topic within doula trainings, largely through the writing and perspectives of Penny Simkin and Phyllis Klaus, who have co-authored a book on this topic.[13] There is debate over whether and how doulas should obtain this information about their clients, much of which has to do with doulas' lack of professional training to deal with any resulting disclosure and implications for the birth experience.

A doula trainer advises helping the woman "see her baby as an ally, not another perpetrator causing pain." She pointed out that the typical hospital method of "purple pushing," which involves instructing a woman to hold her breath and push vigorously as the nurses count down from ten for three cycles, can be traumatic for abuse survivors. However, with physiologic pushing, in which the woman pushes during contractions as she feels like it, breathing normally, the woman does not feel so vulnerable. The trainer warns doulas, "Be careful about language. I get nauseous thinking about it—saying things like, "It'll be over soon, don't fight it," only further immobilizes and disempowers her. Try to say things that help her stay present."

At the postpartum visit, trainees learn that the doula is there to see and admire the baby and hear the woman's story of the birth. Trainers caution the doula to not assume that the woman will agree with the doula's perspective of the birth. One doula trainer gave an example of a woman's birth that was by all objective measures easy and normal. However, the woman told her at the postpartum visit, "I really felt traumatized," and in the ensuing discussion the trainer discovered that she had "felt vulnerable in every way, shape, and form." The trainer learned her client had felt exposed and stripped to her inner core, knowing that she was doing things in the presence of many people that she had previously only done in private: the moaning sounds she used while lovemaking, vomiting, voiding her bladder, and defecating while pushing.

---

13 Interestingly, two recent books on this topic were either self-published or published by a niche press–the topic is one that mainstream presses (academic or trade) seem reluctant to publish, despite the salience and prevalence of the issue for women (Simkin & Klaus, 2004; Sperlich & Seng, 2008).

A trainee responded to this story, wondering if all women feel the same in terms of vulnerability, because, she says nonchalantly, "I didn't care. Maybe it helps to be an exhibitionist." The instructor did not address this comment directly, nor did she provide an explanation as to why the woman in her story had the reaction she described, even with a doula present. Instead, another trainee asked:

If she has mentioned ahead of time her desire for privacy, and then she's in labor, on her hands and knees, genitals exposed, should the doula cover her? Would that respect her desire, or would that action tell the woman there was something to be ashamed of in her behavior when she looks back on the birth?

This question, and the trainer's lack of a definitive answer, points to a dilemma faced by practicing doulas. If anything may have some potentially traumatic, long-lasting impact on the woman's memory of her birth, how can the doula know the consequences of her actions ahead of time?

The diversity of trainees—their backgrounds and prior experience with birth, coupled with the limited time in a typical training, means that complex situations are either left as open questions or given pat solutions. In the above situation, despite an attempt by the trainee to evaluate the extent of the overarching claim—that a woman who is exposed at a birth may carry the scars of her mistreatment forever—the trainer acknowledged the point, then provided an even more extreme example. She related a story about a client who had changed doctors after being inappropriately touched by her male physician: during her birth, despite the woman's written request to not have any men present, this same male physician entered the room and stood against the back wall, arms crossed, watching while the woman pushed. The trainer, as her doula, noticed her client's expression change when this man entered the room. As the doula, however, she felt powerless to do or say anything about this unwelcome intrusion into the labor room. The female physician, however, alert to the situation, confronted her colleague, asking, "Can I help you?" He replied, "Oh, I just wanted to see if I could help." The female physician responded, "We're fine, we can handle it," but had to say this several times before the male physician walked out. After relating this story, the trainer continued to discuss strategies that sexually abused women use to cope with triggers raised during labor and birth.

Trainees learn that a large part of the doula's impact on the woman's memory of birth is accomplished through continuous presence, unconditional support, and reframing events as they happen so as to acknowledge and validate the woman's effort. In the event that the woman feels unhappy or disappointed about some aspect of the birth, the doula's role is to validate her feelings about what happened, but reaffirm choices she made by reminding her of the factors affecting those choices. This reframing activity is a major part of doula training, designed to ensure a "positive birth memory" for the woman, regardless of the doula's opinion or experience of the birth.

From Training to Doula Practice

Doula training workshops are intense, emotional, intellectual, introductory, and contradictory. As the data from one local case study showed (and was confirmed anecdotally by trainers in other geographic locations), a minority (about 30%) of trainees go on to become certified and/or currently practicing doulas (Setubal, 2001). At present, a self-selection process weeds out the unmotivated, disorganized, or otherwise preoccupied trainee. Of the 45 doulas interviewed in my study, only six were not certified. Of these, only one made the deliberate choice to actively practice without certification from any organization; the other five had taken the training within the past year and planned to become certified.

Doulas describe their desire to help other women during birth as a passion or a calling. When asked about her view of birth, Karen Beatty, a retired maternity nurse who transitioned into doula work said:

> How do you talk about something that is just a passion? It's just such an honor to be with someone who we know, but not very well. It's on a professional level, but on an emotional basis too, and it's such a joy to, with a total stranger, be so involved at a most vulnerable time.

Maisy Simmons, who left a well-paying job to become a doula, noted, "The only way to describe this is, it's a calling. I'm not religious ... but this is absolutely something I need to do."

The irony that someone can be so passionate about something that pays so little and takes so much effort is not lost on Judy Dixon, who offers this reason for why women continue to work as doulas after the initial glow and excitement of the work has worn off:

> Yeah, it definitely does take some obsession. I don't know what drives people to it other than obsession. Who wants to be on call 24/7 and stay awake for however long it may take? It's not glamorous. There's very little glamour in it.

Along with their passion for their work, doulas feel birth is a special time; being present at a birth is seen as a great honor regardless of the circumstances. Tiffany Smith says "There's nothing like being there when you can feel the universe open up at the start of a new life."

A major theme in childbirth and new motherhood literature is how women's experience of birth changes their views and awareness of issues in maternity care. While not limited to those who have unmedicated hospital births or homebirths (which are by their nature unmedicated), there is a certain intensity to the experience and how it is talked about afterwards for those who birth without pharmacological pain relief (Gaskin, 1977/1990; Johnson, 1999; Kitzinger, 1989; Klassen, 2001; Oakley, 1979). When asked how they became doulas, many women in this study began their story with their own birth experience, which opened their awareness to the significance of birth. Deborah Rothman said the birth of her child made her realize "this whole other world." She now feels she had been ignorant of this post-birth world, and insensitive to it before she had children. Her reproductive experiences included one abortion and one miscarriage before her first live birth, so her awareness of a "whole other world" came only after giving birth.

Doulas whose first birth experiences were negative often question and conduct research to understand what went wrong. Phyllis Goldman observes:

> You know, I can't even remember how I heard about doulas, but ever since I had two very lonely experiences in childbirth in the 1960s, it kept nagging at me and I thought "there's a better way to do this."

The following birth story from long-time doula, childbirth educator, and author Henci Goer eloquently reflects not only some of the practices that childbirth activists successfully lobbied to eliminate in hospital births, but also the personally transformative effects attributed to an emotionally satisfying birth experience. In response to how she got started as a doula, Henci recalls:

> I had my first child in 1974, although it was an uncomplicated vaginal birth, it was deeply traumatizing. [INT:

In what way?] Well, let's see, in 1974—this is still IVs, enemas, and shaving, heavy-duty narcotics, which I didn't really need, I was talked into that. And then I was talked into a saddle block, which was the dumbest anesthesia going because they didn't give it to you until you are within about ten minutes of giving birth by your own effort, so that they can put you on the delivery table, cut a huge episiotomy, and pull your baby out with forceps. I was tied down to the delivery table. The only thing I can say for it was that my husband was present, and I was conscious. I had terrible problems with the episiotomy. I believe that either he cut an episio-rectomy or it tore, because I had really serious problems afterwards. They showed you the baby. Being tied down on the delivery table, by the way, was very traumatizing, being restrained. They had this new policy where you could nurse the baby in the delivery room, which amounted to them plopping the baby on your chest, telling you, "Now, you don't even want to raise your head, because you've had this spinal," and kind of standing there staring at you while you fumbled around a little, and then they took the baby off to the nursery for a mandatory 12-hour observation period, but since my 12 hours ended at night, they wouldn't bring him to me until the next morning, at which point the warmest I could work up for him was, I thought he was cute. I had severe postpartum depression.

When I got pregnant again—we moved to California when I was six months pregnant—I knew I wanted something very different. I was asking around and I said I wanted a homebirth in the hospital, and they said, "Oh, you want Don Creevy.'" Don is basically an obstetrician who is a midwife. So I spoke with him, and he said, "We have this new policy where you don't go to the delivery room, and no, I never cut episiotomies," and he just sounded like heaven. So I had this terrifically empowering birth, where I had no interventions other than a little fetal monitoring, no medications, it was an unmedicated birth. He helped out her head and shoulders, and then said, "You want the baby? Pull it up." So this is a very powerful moment for me, because it's like a double-exposure negative. I had the memory of instinctively reaching for my son, being restrained by the cuffs on the delivery table, and hearing the doctor say, "Don't touch, this is a sterile field." And overlaid over that is reaching down and lifting out my daughter onto my chest.

So after that birth, I really wanted to get involved in birth. For one thing, I really wanted to attend a birth, and for another, I wanted to be involved in teaching women that the choices they made about their experience really mattered. Because that birth changed my entire feelings about who I was. [INT: How do you think they changed?] Well, I remember she was posterior, so I was okay until I got to pushing, and then it was just unbelievable; it was like someone dropped a truck on my back, but everyone was really encouraging, telling me, "You can do this," and also I hadn't had any medication. I had gotten to a point in labor where I said, "Well, I don't know if I can do this," and everybody around me, instead of saying "Fine, we'll get the drugs," my husband, and the nurse, and Don said, "No, no you can do this, you're almost there"—they encouraged me. And I remember a few days after the birth, I was taking a shower and I was loving my body. And you know, women hate their bodies because we're always too fat or too little on top or too hippy or too whatever, and I was just thinking my body was wonderful.

So it was a transformational experience for me, and I'm not the only other woman who ... if you talk to women who've had this epiphany type of birth, it changes you forever. I'm absolutely clear I would not be who I am today without that birth experience. I think psychologically, it's a matter of accomplishing something that's extremely challenging—so difficult that you're not sure you can do it—is what triggers that transformation. I almost think, because I've done some reading about this, it probably has to involve some physical, not just mental, not just something like passing your bar exam, or something like that. It has to involve a physical challenge for that transformation to occur. You just don't think of yourself in the same way after that (H. Goer, personal communication, January 3, 2002).

Women who have had positive birth experiences often, but not always, turn outward to help other women realize the importance of or achieve a positive birth experience (Bobel, 2002; Davis & Pascali-Bonaro, 2010; Klassen, 2001). Those women who actively educate others about their choices in childbirth, however, often find support from existing childbirth education and midwifery resources within supportive community networks of like-minded women (Lake, Epstein, & Mortiz, 2010). The combined efforts of researching their options, finding a caregiver with whom they could make conscious, informed decisions, and then having a very different experience with subsequent births provides but does not guarantee the desire to become a childbirth activist and advocate for women's birth experiences.

As noted in the training and made central in the recent work of Penny Simkin and Phyllis Klaus on traumatic childbirth, doulas believe birth matters—not just because it has the potential to be a transformational experience leading to a positive re-evaluation of a woman's self-identity, but because it also has the potential to be traumatizing, leading to postpartum depression, relationship difficulties, and other untoward effects. While some of the more egregious practices as Henci Goer and so many other women experienced are no longer routine, there are still ways in which labor management and childbirth practices can be experienced as traumatic. Some, but not all traumatic births may be linked to a woman's sexual abuse history in ways that medical practitioners and even sexual abuse survivors may not realize ahead of time (Simkin & Klaus, 2004; Sperlich & Seng, 2008).

According to a survey conducted on behalf of Washington's Office of Crime Victims Advocacy, 23% of respondents who were randomly contacted for a telephone survey answered "Yes" when asked if they'd ever experienced "sexual penetration by use of force or threat of harm," the state's definition of rape (Birkland & Green, 2001).

Many doulas have seen firsthand how women's sexual abuse histories can affect their birth experiences. About a third of the doulas in this study shared stories connecting sexual abuse and birth experiences. Doula Tiffany Smith said, "Actually, the majority of the women that I've worked with have said 'yes' to that [item on her client questionnaire about sexual abuse]. I think that sexual abuse is a pretty common thing."

Doulas address these issues prenatally if, like Tiffany, they ask women about their history and develop a birth plan specifying that no men other than the woman's partner be present during labor. Sometimes, as in the example provided by the trainer, women's primary care providers may be aware of the issue and support specific requests. Doulas speak about helping women overcome feelings of shame about their bodies and being careful of the language they use at a birth. When obstetric clinicians exhibit insensitive language or behavior, even simply by treating such women's births as routine, the survivor's feelings of physical and emotional disempowerment may resurface during or after their birth experience.[14] Doulas want to ensure that these women in particular are treated with respect and dignity in hospital birth settings.

---

14 There are many complex issues involved when doulas address these experiences with their clients: the lack of professional counseling training; concerns about the propriety of asking clients about sexual abuse history, and whether this is within the doula's scope of practice. These issues deserve further exploration.

Sustaining Doula Practice

Doulas need support to do what they do. They craft a narrative of consequentiality, both medical and emotional, for birthing women and their babies. This claim to a greater good and the sense of doula work as a "calling" stems from deep passion and commitment to supporting women and provides strong internal support for individual women to sustain their doula practice. But the on-call, unpredictable nature of the work, combined with the long hours and low pay (if there is any pay at all) for an emotionally intense experience, while exhilarating, is also exhausting. Maisy Simmons articulates the downside of being on call:

Yeah, I love it. But when I'm waiting for a client to give birth, I really wonder, why on earth am I doing this? What a pain in the butt. We can't go away this weekend. I can't be too far away from my car. I can't go for long walks that take me an hour and a half to get there. I can't go hiking in the mountains because I can't get back in time, and I don't have my equipment. It's just so stressful, because this pager isn't always working, and I don't want to be wired to the hilt and you know, [sighs]. I have to get enough sleep every night. I can't go out and have two or three glasses of wine. I can only have one glass of wine, you know, and that is just a big hassle [smiles ruefully].

In order to manage the uncertain timing and duration of a labor and childbirth, doulas rely on close family members be emotionally supportive and understanding, but also physically present. Only three of the doulas in my study had neither a significant partner nor children. One of these women was the most stressed and over-extended of all the doulas at the time of the interview. In the preceding week, she had had two marathon births—one lasting 45 hours and the other 60 hours. Perhaps if she had children or a partner, she would not have felt she could remain at each of those births for the entire time without calling on her back-up.

Doulas who had significant others spoke of support they provided. Alix Martin relates:

> My boyfriend was so proud of me. Every time I came home from a birth, he'd be like, "Oh, you're so wonderful." It makes him love me more almost, that I'm helping women like this. He thinks it is so wonderful. So that helps.

At the time she was doing those births, they were not yet married. They have since had a child and gotten married. Alix has continued to work as a doula, with her husband's full support. She pumps her breast milk while at births, and if she is away for an extended period, her husband has brought the baby to her at the birth so she can nurse.

Kris Turner has older children, but she also says:

> I have felt very supported—my family has been very understanding of my decision to do this work. It goes back to my husband's experience of birth; he was a wonderful doula, in his way. He was really able to be there, and it just seemed like a natural thing to him that I'd want to do this for other women.

While Alix's boyfriend could imagine and admire the help that Alix was providing other women, Kris attributes her husband's support to his own experience as a doula at her birth. The benefits they each received from their husbands' ability to "be there" made it "natural" for them to understand and support their doing this for others.

Husbands who support their spouses' work assume numerous responsibilities. Doulas speak of husbands who answer phone calls late at night from anxious clients and who have learned enough about birth to reassure the client when they take messages. Mira Godwin tells about her husband overhearing a conversation with her client on the phone, and then afterwards asking her why she didn't tell the client about a particular option that might be of use to her. Mira realized he was right, and called the client back with the information.

Naomi Olsen, a great grandmother, says her retired husband gets a bit impatient when she is gone and used to page her frequently during a birth. Since she had to leave the hospital grounds in order to call him back on her cell phone, this posed a problem. She resolved the matter by telling him that she'll call him as often as she can, and she does. That way he doesn't page her and he still knows what's going on. She notes in a wry, but warm tone, "He loves to pass messages on. Other than that [about the paging], he's very supportive."

Kris Turner's husband is not the only one who has acted as a doula. Debbie Oldham's husband was there for their daughter when she had her babies. Debbie recalls, "He worked those births. The first one, he could not take his hands off her or she would scream. She needed her daddy. He's been there for her constantly. He's got the temperament."

Doula accounts show how doula practice is sustained by husbands who take pride in what their wives are doing and support them not just in spirit, but with practical, hands-on child care, warm meals, and for many a sympathetic audience upon returning home with the story of the birth.

A few doulas said their husbands weren't particularly interested and simply accepted their partner's passion without wanting to hear much about the details.

> He leaves me alone so I can sleep, that's pretty much all I need. Answers the phone if it rings, stuff like that. [INT: He's understanding of what you do?] Oh yeah, he just doesn't want to hear about it, he says, "Don't say placenta in front of me, I don't want to know." So I know I can't

come home and debrief with him, because he doesn't want to hear it ... If I need to gripe, I can always post it on the doula [email] list, then I feel better ... Most of my friends are doulas. It helps a lot, I can talk to any of them about it, and you tend to get immersed in the doula community, because other people don't want to hear about placentas all the time (Stacey Kinney).

Judy Dixon, married and a doula for over 15 years, recounted a revelatory experience her husband had. One day, she casually asked him to admire the camera work in one of her videotaped births. They watched the film together, and he went back to what he had been doing. Judy was surprised when, a few days later, out of the blue:

He just said, "You know, I just totally see what it is you're doing in a completely different light right now. It's like God's work. It's like karma bonus points up the wazoo. You're banking this incredible amount of karma by just helping these people through birth." And I hadn't really ever seen it in that light before. Religious people talk about service, as a means to their faith, as a path to their God or whatever, but basically that's what this is too, we have these little banks out there that we're banking some good karma by doing this. [She paused as though to reflect.] It was a good birth. [INT: He's been with you through how many years of you doing this, did a light kind of flash?] All along it was more, "Oh, she's at a birth, I have to be child responsible," that was more what it was all about as opposed to what I was really doing (Judy Dixon).

Judy's work as a doula had remained hidden from view, so her husband had seen it primarily as a demand for (his) increased parental responsibilities when she was away. Seeing her work on the video provided a new lens for him to acknowledge the larger meaning within her work—"God's work" or "karma bonus points"—that even she hadn't considered before.

While spouses may understand and support the doula's passion, children can be less accepting of the idea that their mother is going off to care for someone else. Emmie Ward laughs when she talks about her sons' feelings about her work: "Well, they've always known me as that person who would sometimes have to leave. So they came to expect it, I guess." Wren George says her daughter really enjoys hearing about the babies, but sometimes the kids complain about her leaving at night or not being there in the morning when they get ready for school. Wren and her doula partner Danna Capelli watch each other's children while the other is at a birth. They also arrange their schedules so that they don't teach childbirth classes or take any doula clients who would be due in the three weeks before and after Christmas or in July and August, when they take family vacations—made possible, they remind their children—by their doula income.

Children benefit from their mothers' work as a doula in ways beyond the additional treats made possible from the income. Several doulas with older children felt that their kids had more knowledge of birth and birth control than most of their peers. Cynthia Lynn takes great satisfaction that her son, in his early 20s, is the only one of his high school friends who has not yet fathered a child. She attributes this to his early and constant awareness growing up that sex has real and long-lasting consequences: pregnancy, birth, and babies.

Kris Turner said one of the benefits to her children is seeing their mother go out and return to them with feelings "that just makes you want to gather them up." These emotions are mixed. In part, the feelings reflect doulas' gratitude to their families for supporting them and understanding why they are doulas, but they are also a response to the sharp contrast between the emotional intensity at a birth with relative strangers and the close connection the doula feels upon returning to the comfort of her own family, heightened by the oxytocin rush she receives from the birth.

The challenges and dilemmas of doula practice provide strong impetus for women to engage in local or online support networks with other doulas. During the time they were attending births, all the doulas in my study were fairly active in local doula organizations or participated in online discussion boards, email listserves, or support groups with other doulas. Most had at least one committed back-up doula partner. All named other doulas as important sounding boards for listening to them share the frustrations, triumphs, and details of their client's births.

Women who do not actively practice, but intend someday to start or resume doula work still have a place in the doula world; they feel part of the community, but are likely to have other family or life commitments. No doula ever renounced the ideology, much like the phrase in midwifery, "once a midwife, always a midwife." As they continue doula work, many women move into allied childbirth fields that offer more professional status, better income, and stable work.

One local trainer in an East coast setting told me that she finds most of her doula trainees become childbirth educators rather than come from their ranks in the first place as many did in the early years of doula training (R.E. Weiss, personal communication, January 27, 2002). Other doulas enroll in midwifery or nursing school to further their interest in technical aspects of maternity care, as well as increase their earning potential. Those who came to doula practice from another field, such as social work or counseling, continue to work in those domains but find their newfound doula experience enhances their professional skills and empathy.

Particular structural, economic, and cultural foundations are essential for women to successfully work as doulas. These include a secure income from another source, whether a husband, a flexible job(s), or retirement benefits. It takes passion, commitment, and a great deal of communication to enlist the support and understanding of family members to undertake the emotional and financial liabilities of women working as doulas.

In addition, by delegating their own family caregiving responsibilities when clients call, doulas demonstrate how other, unknown women's birth experiences take priority over everything else. Children learn that there are others whose needs take priority in their mothers' lives. Spouses or babysitters assume full responsibility for their children within the limited timeframe the doula is away. After the birth, the doula returns to the everyday, a place where the practical work of caring is infrequently acknowledged or appreciated by those who take that work and the woman who provides it for granted.

The typical practicing doula, then, is a woman who has been drawn by passion to provide care to other women during their births. She has adopted a belief in the transformative and empowering effects of unmedicated, low-intervention childbirth, but also in the right and ability of women to make their own choices. She strives to provide education and information to women that will give them an open mind to experience whatever lies in store for them at their births. She networks intensively with others who share her beliefs and help her attain her goals. The lifestyle is hard to maintain. Ideology, rather than professional status or economic reward, keeps the doula going with the conviction that she is changing the world and making a difference.

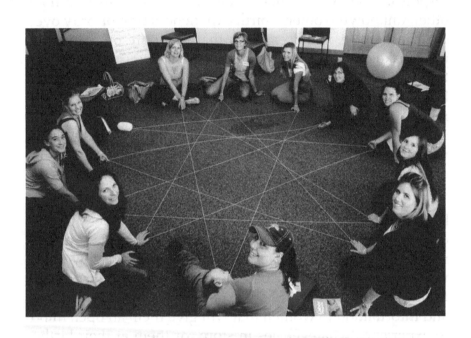

Photo 12. Doulas at the close of a training workshop: "We weave a web of sisterly support ... promising to doula each other as we doula the motherbaby and her family."
Photo by Kyndal May.

Personal Story

THE GUIDE
Kelly Martineau

The room is dim, the time just after midnight. Dawn seems but a distant dream. A few hours into active labor, I know I will not sleep tonight.

My body tightens into contraction every five minutes. While a nurse monitors the baby's heartbeat, I lie on my back on the hospital bed, unable to fold into the sitting position that has made labor manageable. My lower back aches, the pain edging into the space between active contractions.

The door opens, and Alissa, my birth doula, enters the room. Her auburn hair is pulled back from her face, and she walks toward me with a calm smile. Her palms gently ease onto my feet. Through my socks, I can feel the warmth of her hands. She cradles my soles with gentle pressure.

As the next contraction begins, I close my eyes and breathe deeply. Through the pain, I feel the strength of Alissa's hands, drawing my attention and energy, rooting me in my body. When the contraction ends, I relax into her care.

Alissa had been grounding me through the final weeks of pregnancy. Each time I called to report possible pre-labor symptoms, she responded calmly. "Yes, it sounds like your body is getting ready," she would say. "You could begin labor tonight or in a few weeks."

During a check-up three days before my due date, the midwife reinforced my certainty that labor was imminent. Due to the baby's station and the degree of dilation, she said she would be surprised if I made it to my due date. When I called Alissa, she remained cautious, repeating her mantra, "It sounds like your body is getting ready."

This calm reassurance was the reason my husband and I had hired Alissa. I decided early in my pregnancy that I wanted a doula to support my labor. As I researched local practitioners, I envisioned a warm, nurturing presence, like that of a grandmother. I pictured the doula enveloping me with kindness, massaging my back, softening the blows of the contractions.

What I first noted about Alissa was her precision. She asked many questions of us, and she responded to our inquiries with clear, comprehensive answers. My husband and I interviewed a second candidate, the epitome of the gentle presence I sought. However, her vague responses left me wanting. Alissa was the clear choice.

Despite the midwife's confident pronouncement, I was still pregnant on Monday, the day after my due date. Alissa checked with me each day by phone until Friday, when my body began the rhythmic contractions of early labor. After my water broke at 11:00 p.m., we left for the hospital, where Alissa joined us.

My eyelids rise, and the world reappears. I see my husband on the periphery, ready to support me. I have moved from the bed to a birthing tub. Although I do not know the time, I sense that hours have passed. The contractions have become so intense that I disconnect from the outside world, shunning knowledge of any metric—time or dilation—that might tell me at which stage of labor I am.

While my back and lower pelvis constrict with each contraction, I feel very little in my abdomen. Alissa tells me that the baby is facing my side and suggests various positions to encourage her to turn toward my back. As the baby's tiny body grates against my bones, I envision my pelvis as a bowl that may crack.

Although I am floating in a birth tub, the buoyant water does little to lift my spirits or the pressure in my back. The pain no longer ebbs between contractions. No matter the position, my lower back aches with the burden of this responsibility. With each contraction, the world around me falls away. There is only force and pain.

And Alissa. I focus on her brown eyes, which never waver in their confidence. Her voice is smooth and sure, as she deflects my protests with encouraging words. I cling to the edge of the tub, and she covers my hands with hers. When I want only to retreat into nothingness, she gently, but firmly, tethers me to my own strength.

I hear murmurs, but I do not wake. I float up to consciousness and let myself drift back to sleep several times before finally opening my eyes. The sun shines on the nearby buildings through cool fall air. It is now early afternoon.

The events of the morning flood my mind. By the last exam, around 6:00 a.m., the baby had turned face up instead of down, meaning that my back labor would continue. In addition, the midwife reported that a small portion of the cervical lip, which had not dissolved, was swelling, and she told me not to push. An hour of fighting that visceral urge siphoned my remaining energy, and, although I had intended a natural birth, I finally requested an epidural. After seven hours of feeling so intensely, I welcomed the spreading numbness that would allow my body to rest.

I am now awake after two hours of sleep. The midwife conducts another exam, and reports with a smile that the baby has turned and descended. It is time to push. Lacking sensation in my legs and pelvis, I wonder how. I know the muscles are not paralyzed, but they seem distant. Recalling how it felt to push from the early morning hours, I focus on my pelvis, trying to activate my body with my mind. Alissa and the midwife applaud my efforts, but after 30 minutes, they feel I need to make more progress.

"Kelly, the baby needs to make her way under your pelvic bone," says Alissa. "Can you visualize her sliding underneath as you push?" She mimics the movement with her hands, one moving under the other like a boat rolling down the trough of a wave.

I focus my energy in the numb basin of my pelvis. As I flex the muscles, I imagine the baby gliding underneath the arcing pelvic bone.

"Wow, that's great!" exclaims the midwife.

"Good, Kelly," says Alissa with a smile. "Just keep focusing on that image."

But I don't need them to tell me it's working. I feel the energy radiating from my pelvis. I can't feel the contractions or the baby, but I can sense her progress, and my body's very real ability to birth.

My husband holds my hand and my gaze. Alissa cradles my bent leg so I can push my foot against a bar for leverage, her support anchoring me to the process as I bring my daughter closer and closer.

After two hours, I make one final push, and my daughter enters the world. With the same vitality she displayed in the womb, she kicks and cries. The midwife delivers her directly to my chest. Her newborn body is warm against my skin. The umbilical cord is still attached, but its pulse slows. The lifeline that had fed her for forty weeks is ceasing to function.

Alissa gently guides me as Ruby nuzzles at my skin. With a soft voice, she helps us negotiate the first feeding. After allowing my husband and me a few minutes alone with our daughter, Alissa ushers our parents and siblings into the room. She plans to leave us in the care of our families and the nurses.

I want her to stay, to enjoy this new life that she has guided into the world. I want her to teach me to feed my daughter. But, save for a few postpartum meetings, her role in our lives is complete. Now, it is my job to nourish, to root this new being to the earth and to her own strength.

Alissa slips quietly out of the room. I hold my daughter in my arms, and we stare at each other through newly opened eyes.

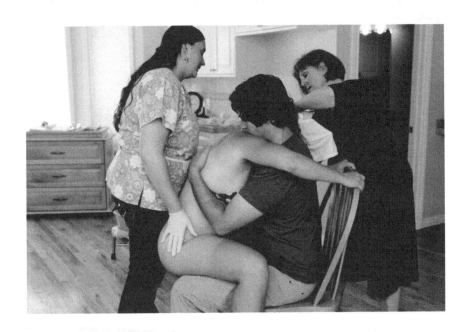

Photo 13. Doula and midwife assisting the laboring woman and her partner in a supported lap pose.
Photo by Kyndal May.

Chapter Three

Mothering the Mother: Trained Professional or Caring Woman?[1]

The world turns to women for mothering, and this fact silently attaches itself to many a job description.

Arlie Russell Hochschild[2]

As doulas establish their occupational niche in maternity care, their claims to professional status are based primarily on organizational standards of practice and certification by any one of a number of organizations currently training and certifying doulas.[3] Doulas assert specialized knowledge of the complex intersection of emotional, physical, and medical aspects of childbirth, yet portray themselves as kind, caring women with a natural, intuitive ability to improve clinical outcomes in medicalized settings. These claims to professional status are complicated by several factors. Sociologists define a profession as a group that controls entry into its own ranks and possesses specialized knowledge verified through

---

1 This chapter is based on the author's sociological research on the history and experiences of doulas in the United States. The methodology is described in the Appendix.

2 Hochschild, A. R. (1983). *The managed heart: Commercialization of human feeling.* Berkeley, CA: University of California Press, p. 170.

3 At present there are at least five national organizations that train and certify doulas.

credentialing and licensing. Admission to the profession, thus, is strictly controlled through organizational means. In contrast, anyone can call himself or herself a doula: it is an unlicensed occupation. Further, the doula's claim to specialized knowledge is largely experiential and rests on the constructed, collective experience as women who have birthed socially, among women, since "the beginning" (Trevathan, 1987).

Aspiring doulas are said to possess "special skills," but also "natural talent," as the founders of DONA International note in their text *Mothering the Mother*, which is on the required reading list of most doula training workshops.

> Women who have the interest and develop the special skills to become a doula may come from a variety of backgrounds ... childbirth educators, lay midwifery ... Some women seem to have a natural bent for the whole process, just as some people are born with perfect pitch, and they seek a role in which to support this talent (Klaus, Kennell, & Klaus, 1993, p. 135).

This chapter examines the dilemmas posed by the juxtaposition of specialized knowledge, the medical and psychological consequentiality of how women are treated during their births, and the claim that a kind, caring woman can accomplish positive impact by intuition alone. These dilemmas create challenges for individual doulas and their organizations. Most critically, the effect of framing doula skills as natural or intuitive is to obscure the real skills, talents, and value of what doulas accomplish.

The Trouble with Research: Clinical Trials on Doula Effectiveness

The paradox of simultaneously being a trained professional and caring woman is present in the randomized control trials on labor support. The scientific "discovery" of the doula's impact on labor and birth outcomes was almost accidental. As noted earlier, researchers Marshall Klaus and John Kennell were interested in how mothers interacted with their premature newborn infants and explored interventions with the potential to positively impact mother-infant bonding. Labor support was not a particular focus in the original pilot study carried out in Guatemala. However, one of the research assistants could not help offering emotional support and encouragement to women as they labored, in addition to her role of observing and recording data.

The researchers subsequently discovered that this continuous emotional support during labor had positive medical outcomes in addition to their primary outcome of interest: enhanced mother-infant bonding. The results, published in 1980 in *The New England Journal of Medicine*, were relatively modest: women who had a doula present had significantly shorter labors and engaged in significantly more interaction with their infants (stroking, smiling, talking) during an observation period. However, the suggestive and unexpected finding that "the likelihood of development of certain problems that require intervention during labor and delivery was lower for mothers who had a supportive companion" spurred the researchers to continue their investigation. From the start, the "doula" was described as "an untrained lay woman" who supported the young Guatemalan women throughout labor and delivery. Support consisted of "physical contact (e.g., rubbing the mother's back and holding her hands), conversation, and the presence of a friendly companion whom the mother had not met before" (Sosa, Kennell, Robertson, & Urrutia, 1980, p. 597).

Another trial took place at a U.S. hospital and was expanded to include more participants, all first-time mothers (Kennell, Klaus, McGrath, Robertson, & Hinkley, 1991). The researchers randomly assigned 412 healthy women in labor with their first baby to a supported group (n = 212) that received the continuous support of a doula or to an observed group (n = 200) that was monitored by a woman who "who never spoke to the laboring woman and attempted to remain as inconspicuous as possible in the midst of the large number of labor room personnel" (p. 2198). A third group, of two hundred four women, were selected for comparison with the supported and observed groups, and assigned to a control group after delivery. A major motivation for conducting this investigation was its potential for reducing high cesarean rates at the Jefferson Davis Hospital in Houston, Texas, a public hospital providing care for a low-income Hispanic, black, and white population (p. 2197). The mean age of laboring women in this study was 20 years, most (80 - 85%) of whom had not attended childbirth education classes—and had on average about 9.5 years of education. Over 65% did not speak English, 50% were single, and most were quite poor (under $15,000 annual income). The patients received care from the staff service (English speaking residents) "who followed established obstetric protocol." Typical conditions under which women labored included a 12-bed ward, "with insufficient privacy to allow visitors," "usually in the presence of strangers." Interpreters were available if needed. The women were "asked to participate in the study after they were admitted to the hospital in active labor" (p. 2197).

The doulas used in this study were required to be fluent in both Spanish and English. They participated in a three-week training session and met daily with each other, and weekly with the investigators, "to ensure a degree of consistency in their methods of supporting patients," and were paid by research funds on an hourly basis for an average of $200 per patient. Doulas first met women after hospital admission, provided emotional, physical and informational support, and "also kept a written record of staff contacts, interventions, and procedures" (pp. 2197-2198). The researchers were surprised by the findings that outcomes improved in both the supported and the observed groups as compared to the control group. Doula trainers emphasize this latter finding in reassuring trainees that as new doulas, their mere presence and kind attention will most assuredly have a positive effect.

These research findings generated additional interest in the potential medical and economic benefits of the presence of a continuous labor support person, whether lay or professional. Subsequent studies have been conducted in South Africa, Finland, Canada, Mexico, Botswana, Belgium, France, Greece, Australia, Brazil, Chile, Nigeria, Sweden, Thailand, and the United States under widely varying hospital and social conditions. The Cochrane Collaboration Pregnancy and Childbirth Group Module has published several reviews of the randomized controlled trials that compare continuous support during labor with usual care. The person providing continuous support in these trials could have been a healthcare professional (midwife or nurse), someone with training as a doula or childbirth educator, or a member of the woman's social network (family, spouse/partner, or friend), or someone with little to no special training in labor support.

The first review, published in 1999, involved 14 trials, and just over 5,000 women while the most recent review, published in 2012, included an evaluation of 22 trials involving more than 15,000 women (Hodnett, 1999; Hodnett, Gates, Hofmeyr, & Sakala, 2012). In 11 of these trials, laboring women were permitted to have family members present; in the other 11 trials, hospital policy excluded family support. Epidural analgesia was not routinely available in seven of the trials, was made routinely available in 14 trials, and the availability of epidural analgesia was unknown in one trial. The findings of this most recent meta-analysis included:

Women who received continuous labour support were more likely to give birth "spontaneously," i.e., give birth with neither caesarean nor vacuum nor forceps. In addition, women were less likely to use pain medications, were more likely to be satisfied, and had slightly shorter labours. Their babies were less likely to have low five-minute Apgar scores. No adverse effects were identified. We conclude that all women should have continuous support during labour. Continuous support from a person who is present solely to provide support, is not a member of the woman's social network, is experienced in providing labour support, and has at least a modest amount of training, appears to be most beneficial. In comparison with having no companion during labour, support from a chosen family member or friend appears to increase women's satisfaction with their childbearing experience. [Furthermore], continuous support during labour has clinically meaningful benefits for mothers and infants and no known harm. All women should have support throughout labor and birth (Hodnett, Gates, Hofmeyr, & Sakala, 2012, p. 2).

The overall effects in each of the outcomes, while significant, are much lower than those found in the earliest doula trials, which can be illustrated by calculating the Relative Risks of particular outcomes among the intervention and control groups of each trial. [A relative risk (RR) of 1 means there is no difference in risk between the two groups.] The 2012 Cochrane Review found that women with continuous labor support were slightly more likely to have a spontaneous vaginal birth (RR 1.08, 95% confidence interval (CI) 1.04 to 1.12), and slightly less likely (RR 0.90, 95% CI 0.84 to 0.96) to have intrapartum analgesia. Although the relative risks are small, the potential for labor support to make a noticeable difference in outcomes may be seen when doulas are present at a large number of births. Currently, the number of births with a doula present is not large enough in any one facility or area to be able to demonstrate a noticeable population-level difference.

In each of these studies, the support provided was characterized as experienced females. "Experience," however, varied from training as a nurse or midwife, doula, or childbirth educator to personal experience with childbirth. Thus, one solution to the problem of medicalized and costly interventions engendered by high technology in impersonal institutions was articulated as the emotional and physical labor of a caring woman, described variously as a "labor companion" (Kennell, Klaus, McGrath, Robertson & Hinkley, 1991); a "supportive companion," "female companion," or "constant human support" (Klaus, Kennell, Robertson, & Sosa, 1986); a "supportive lay woman ("doula") (Sosa, Kennell, Robertson, & Urrutia, 1980), at much lower cost to hospitals than trained professionals (Tew, 1998).

Nurses and the Provision of Labor Support

Researcher and nurse Ellen Hodnett provides an important, critical perspective on the issue of labor support provided by professional nurses versus doulas. Her research on the effects of labor support has been motivated by her allegiance to nursing, but complicated by her recognition of women's needs in childbirth. She writes:

> As a nurse, I worry about the future of the profession if nurses relinquish the clearly effective aspects of their care to less-skilled workers. As a woman, however, I wonder if it matters who provides the support, as long as it is provided (Hodnett, 1997, p. 79).

Research findings are mixed in terms of the effect of labor support provided by professional nurses or midwives on childbirth outcomes (Gagnon & Waghorn, 1996; Gagnon, Waghorn, & Covell, 1997; Hodnett, 1997; Hodnett, Lowe, Hannah, & Gagnon, 2003). Exploring possible reasons for why trained nurses have been found to be less effective as labor support providers raises important issues for future research. Some work-sampling studies point to the reduced time that nurses spend physically touching laboring patients (Gagnon & Waghorn, 1996; Korst, Eusebio-Angeja, Chamorro, Aydin, & Gregory, 2003; McNiven, Hodnett, & O'Brien-Pallas, 1992).

Reasons for why labor support provided by nurses is less effective are as yet unsubstantiated in research. However, Hodnett points to a nursing culture of care in which peers disapprove of nurses who spend too much time with the laboring woman, despite the clear medical benefits associated with hands-on care (Hodnett, 1997). Nurses may not provide physical support due to several factors: among them, a lack of training on non-pharmacological methods of pain relief, the near universal use of epidurals, and/or the subsequent devaluation of emotional care in their hospital maternity units.

In 2011, I attended a conference at which coordinators from a health maintenance organization described a quality-improvement project initiated in the labor and delivery unit in order to increase patient satisfaction scores. Nurses in the unit were asked to approach a laboring woman at her bedside, sit down, and make eye and physical contact when introducing themselves. The project coordinators described how astounded they were by the resistance from the nurses to change their practice. The coordinators identified three objections from nurses about this proposed change: fears that women would not like this behavior, doubts in their ability to accomplish the actions successfully, and being unconvinced this approach would make a difference. Once these barriers were overcome, however, the resulting increase in patient satisfaction surprised the nurses and they quickly became champions of the approach. Such an outcome would likely not surprise doulas or others who recognize the value and impact of high touch in healthcare settings. The nurses' resistance speaks to the changes many observers have seen in American hospital birth environments, where "institutional routines, high rates of intervention, unfamiliar personnel, lack of privacy, and other conditions that may be experienced as harsh" (Hodnett, Gates, Hofmeyr, & Sakala, 2012, p. 3).

The Problem with Statistics in Promoting Labor Support

In the early years of doula organizational growth, the statistics supporting the benefits of continuous labor support were widely cited and continue to be used in promotional materials, such as brochures, websites, and books about the benefits of doulas. However, at least three problems emerged with this early strategy to justify and promote the doula role at births. The first stems from the fallacious reasoning of applying generalized statistical outcomes to particular events: the ecological fallacy. The second problem concerns the qualitatively different contexts in which the studies were conducted (i.e., public hospitals, developing countries) from those in which most American doulas work. Finally, in the past decade, birth outcomes in the U.S. have worsened for both mothers and babies with record rates of cesarean deliveries. Taken as a whole, many women feel they have failed as doulas when their clients experience highly interventive, medicalized births.

The randomized clinical trials on the effectiveness of the doula role may have legitimized the idea of doula care within some medical settings, highlighted as a selling point for hospital-based volunteer doula programs or viewed instrumentally as a way to increase patient satisfaction scores, which are now frequently tied to insurance reimbursements. However, in other ways, the clinical trials have proved detrimental to individual doula practice; over time these outcomes have not been realized for most women in the American context (Block, 2007; Gordon, Walton, McAdam, Derman, Gallitero, & Garrett, 1999). Midwife and author Pam England, creator of *Birthing from Within*, a Zen-inspired revisioning of childbirth education, addressed this issue in an essay directed to doulas

(England, 2000). She argues that current childbirth education focuses too much on rational information and not enough on women's intuitive knowledge of how to give birth.

> I'm especially concerned when I see people carrying their intentions to re-create the impressive statistics about the difference doulas can make in labor. While research plays an important role in penetrating the awareness of birthing families and institutions, its value in one context can be a detriment in another moment. In a culture obsessed with measuring and controlling birth outcome, doulas are at risk of being caught up, albeit with good intentions, in an outcome-based mindset. Focusing on outcome makes it difficult for parents and doulas to labor in the moment ... I know of too many doulas who felt helpless and discouraged when, in spite of all their efforts and long hours, they could not make "enough" difference. Mother after mother was induced, or labors did not unfold naturally; birth after birth was medicalized. For many dedicated doulas, the feeling of loss become so great, they simply quit being doulas (England, 2000).

Pam England's prescription for this problem is not to educate doulas on the dangers of the ecological fallacy or point out the situational and cultural differences between women and hospital policies in the studies and the typical doula client in U.S. hospitals. Rather, she encourages doulas to come to births "empty-handed and open-hearted," adopting a mindset she calls "birthing in awareness."

During the course of my research in the late 1990s and early 2000s, only a few doulas critiqued the use of these statistics and expressed concern that so many doulas were quoting them in brochures, and perhaps misleading client expectations about what the doula fee might save them in terms of hospital costs. Jodi Park is one who opposed their use in advertising doula services.

They [statistics] give people the idea there will be magic. It sets up unrealistic expectations on the part of the clients. If the doctor has a 65% c-section rate, the doula doesn't have that much control over it. Women [doula clients] can end up feeling hurt and betrayed.

In 1999, the time of this interview, few doulas shared this concern. Jodi continues by elaborating how statistics obscure what she thinks is the main goal for doulas.

Some people believe that the doula's job is to prevent c-sections or epidurals. That should not be our goal. Our goal is that the woman has a satisfactory experience, she's empowered through it, as a strong, capable, competent person, and that this transfers over to her role as mother.

In the next couple of years, however, the emphasis on the doula's impact on birth outcomes began to shift within major doula organizations. At the 2000 DONA conference, Marshall Klaus presented a lecture on a recent European research study that did not show dramatic medical benefits to supported births. Klaus pointed out differences in U.S. and European childbirth philosophy, practice, and attendants, and introduced new research exploring the effects of doula care on postpartum adjustment and outcomes. He noted that little attention had been given to the doula's impact on mother-infant interaction, the original focus of the early clinical trials, and outlined some of the preliminary findings and ongoing research in this area by his pediatrician colleague Dr. John Kennell. When asked about this shift during our 2001 interview, Debbie Young, then -editor of the DONA's newsletter, *International Doula,* and chair of the Third-Party Reimbursement Committee recounted the discussion at the 2001 DONA conference in Milwaukee.

Presenters at the conference stressed that original statistics are history. New positive studies have been done, but even those you can't apply across the board. The strongest message to that effect in my recollection from the conference was that we're not talking about numbers—we are talking about people. They really were trying to communicate this. Numbers are not what we're about. This is a shift, in the last three years more slowly, but very strong at this last conference. Let's get away from numbers and focus on what we can do for people. For the common doula (without statistics education), the numbers seem very impressive. I understand that desire to use the numbers. I've been a doula trainer since 1994. I've shifted away from using numbers in my training. (D. Young, personal communication, December 12, 2001).

While the Cochrane meta-analysis found no negative effects for providing continuous emotional, physical, and informational support to women in labor, there is little evidence that continuous labor support provided by doulas has a significant positive impact in all practice settings. One study excluded from the Cochrane Review for methodological reasons was conducted in an HMO hospital in Northern California, and found that labor support from doulas had a desirable effect on epidural use (54.4% versus 66.1%, p< .05), and women's perceptions of birth, but did not alter need for operative deliveries (Gordon, Walton, McAdam, Derman, Gallitero, & Garrett, 1999, p. 422).

In another trial with professional nurse-*monitrices* providing continuous labor support, key outcomes, such as use of oxytocin, epidural, forceps, and cesarean section, were not different among women in the two groups (Hodnett & Osborn, 1989b). However, a comment on that study noted that the practice habits of obstetricians may have "utterly swamped any effect of added support during labor and delivery" (Shearer, 1989, p. 183).

In contrast, Shearer notes, the trials reviewed in another study by Boylan (1989) did control for individual obstetrician's practice habits by having them all agree at the outset to a clear, uniform protocol for why and how each procedure is done. Without such agreement in the American obstetrics community, however, individual doula efforts to impact key outcomes, especially cesarean rates, with their clients' births are unlikely to succeed.

Cesarean Delivery Rates and Doulas

The initial optimism doulas felt about their ability to make a difference in U.S. birth outcomes has been dampened by several factors. The increased rates of interventions, particularly cesarean section rates, have been accompanied by studies showing most women (83%) are relatively satisfied with the care they received during their birth hospitalization (Declercq, Sakala, Corry, Applebaum, & Herrlich, 2013). Doulas, while a promising intervention, are merely a drop in the birth bucket, and nationally representative surveys have shown the percent of U.S. births with a doula present remained fairly steady over the past decade, at 5% in 2002; 3% in 2006, and 6% in 2012. This translates into about 201,086, 127,979, and 237,125 women who had doulas in each of the three survey periods.[4]

The overall medical community's response to the early studies and to doula support is difficult to assess (Eftekhary, Klein, & Xu, 2010). While promoters and organizers of hospital-based doula programs use outcome data as a way to convince hospital administrators to support such initiatives, they acknowledge that many such programs are driven by the ef-

---

4 In 2002, there were 4,021,726 live births; in 2006, 4,265,996 and in 2011, the most recent year available at this time, 3,953,593. Source: Department of Health and Human Services, National Center for Health Statistics, web: http://www.cdc.gov/nchs/births.htm. Accessed 5/13/13.

forts of one champion and if that person leaves, the program often falters. Although one evaluation of a hospital-based doula program found positive benefits (Deitrick & Draves, 2008), overall cuts to public health funding for maternal-child programs throughout the mid-2000s left little room for expanding services in this area.

Recently, however, provisions in the Affordable Care Act ("ObamaCare") have opened the door to Medicaid funding for community doula programs, and several initiatives are underway across the country to increase low-income women's access to doula care. Some cost-benefit analyses show economic savings to states if doula-attended births had lower rates of cesarean sections (Kozhimannil, Hardeman, Attanasio, Blauer-Peterson, & O'Brien, 2013), although others have questioned the ethical and practical issues of paying doulas less than $250 to $300 to achieve such cost-savings (Morton & Basile, 2013).

Cesarean rates are influenced by a complex set of drivers and constraints that operate at the individual, hospital, and state levels. Variation in state and hospital rates, as well as facility-level policies and protocols affecting clinical practice have all been shown to play a role. Proposing the doula as a bandage to what many in the maternity world see as a gaping wound (a 33% cesarean delivery rate) won't address this underlying systemic problem. A policy approach that neglects obstetricians, nurses, and hospitals in ongoing quality improvement efforts to reduce non-medically indicated cesareans, and instead focuses on the underpaid, least-valued member of the team—the doula—may be less likely to succeed in its goal to improve maternity outcomes. Furthermore, finding the necessary number of qualified doulas who are able to provide labor support at the economic level that would result in cost savings may be problematic (Morton & Basile, 2013). A more complete understanding of the factors involved in the high rate of cesarean births is needed before doulas or other labor support persons are offered as the low-cost answer

(Main, Morton, Hopkins, Giuliani, Melsop, & Gould, 2011; Morris, 2013; Sleutel, 2000).

It is crucial that policy discussions focused on improving maternity care bear in mind that high cesarean rates are primarily a problem of obstetric culture and practice. The solution to this problem needs to involve reforming obstetric practices from within and cannot rest wholly on the shoulders of doulas. The most recent Cochrane Collaboration report on doula care points out that in addition to doula support, if reductions in cesarean rates are to occur:

> Changes to the content of health professionals' education and to the core identity of professionals may also be important. Policy makers and administrators must look at system reform and rigorous attention to evidence-based use of interventions that were originally developed to diagnose or treat problems and are now used routinely during normal labours (Hodnett, Gates, Hofmeyr, & Sakala, 2012, p. 16).

Doula Care in the Postpartum Period

Beyond reducing cesarean rates, another claim for doula care is that "mothering the mother" results in better psychological adjustment postpartum. An early study examining this issue looked at first-time mothers' working models of caregiving, and compared women who received doula support with those who received typical Lamaze preparation for birth (childbirth classes). The study was based on interviews with 35 predominantly white, middle-class, first-time mothers in the third trimester, and again at four months postpartum. The interviews focused on "feelings about being a mother, the imagined (prebirth) or actual (postbirth) relationship with the child, and imagined (prebirth) or actual (postbirth) separations" (Manning-Orenstein, 1998, p. 75). The interviews were coded and rated on four scales: rejecting, uncertain, secure, and helpless.

> Mothers in the doula group were significantly less reject-
> ing and helpless in their working models of caregiving
> than were the mothers in the Lamaze group. In addition,
> the women in the doula group were less emotionally dis-
> tressed and had higher self-esteem ... and rated their in-
> fants as significantly less fussy than the mothers in the La-
> maze group (p. 73).

Both groups in this study described their birth experiences similarly, suggesting that the doula's presence does not shield birthing women from negative encounters with their doc-tors or hospital procedures. However, this similarity between groups "adds support to the argument that the more positive outcomes for the mothers in the doula group resulted from the presence of the doula" (p. 79).

Manning-Orenstein is a licensed marriage, family, and child counselor who locates the doula within the therapeu-tic realm. She argues the "holding environment" created by the doula's presence is "similar to what occurs in therapy. The conditions of therapy are present: the close alliance be-tween mother and doula, the mother's heightened receptivity to change, the reinforcement of her positive attributes, and the practicing of new behaviors" (p. 80). The focus in Man-ning-Orenstein's study is an explicit evaluation of individu-al women's mothering and nurturing behaviors within the theoretical paradigm of attachment theory. The study's find-ings are necessarily limited due to the small sample size and non-random assignment of women to each group. The author ends with a discussion of famed psychoanalyst D.W. Winn-icott's observation:

> When maternal care is going well, it is scarcely noticed.
> In other words, good mothering is all but invisible ... Ob-

serving mothers at birth who are well supported in doing what comes naturally helps to reestablish our faith in this invisible maternal capability (p. 80).

The Invisibility of Good Care

The invisibility of "good" mothering as well as good caregiving in gendered occupations, such as childcare, nursing, and elder care has been well documented (Gordon, Benner, & Noddings, 1996; Hochschild, 1983). The doula's contribution to postpartum psychological adjustment is an important area for further research, as are more sociologically informed and oriented analyses of the interactions between medical caregivers and birthing women and new mothers and their babies. Too often, the natural rhetoric of birthing advocates minimizes the skill and effort required to provide effective doula care and support to a laboring woman in the midst of a highly technical and medicalized birth setting. This has the unfortunate effect of assuming that good doula care, like good mothering, comes naturally and without effort.

The practical achievement of effective doula care is nevertheless a product of skill and communication. Maisy Simmons's story illustrates how new doulas feel anxious and uncertain in their abilities to provide labor support given their awareness of the consequentiality of women's labor experiences to their physical and emotional well-being. Maisy was referred to her first client, an Ethiopian Muslim woman, by a more experienced doula who needed a backup. When she met her client prenatally very close to her due date, Maisy got the impression that the pregnant woman "wasn't interested in childbirth, she didn't really care." At that prenatal visit, Maisy mentioned that her doula care during labor would involve touching her client's body in places where Maisy perceived tension. The woman's job, said Maisy, was to concentrate on getting rid of tension in those places the doula touched. Maisy had little time to worry about her upcoming performance, as she was called unexpectedly to the hospital very soon after this first and only visit. Maisy recalls her feelings at the time:

> I was really nervous before I got there, but it was good that I didn't have a lot of warning because I just had to go and do it. I remembered what they said at training was "All you need to do is be there—if you are just there it improves the outcome, anything you add on top of that is just a plus." Fine, I thought, I can be there.

Maisy's dilemma about what she would do as a first-time doula gets at the heart of the contradictions within doula care. The training is brief, there is no supervised student learning, the mode of care can be merely touching a body, but the outcomes are said to be medically and emotionally consequential for the laboring woman. Maisy made the commitment to just "be there." She described the birth as very satisfactory for her client, who labored after a Pitocin induction and gave birth to her first child without any pain medications. Maisy continues with her story:

> Yeah, she did it. She had no drugs, did the whole thing naturally, and I was amazed. She thought it was great, and she said she'd never in her life been as relaxed as she was in labor! [INT: You wouldn't normally think that's a time of the greatest relaxation]. I wouldn't! [Laughter]. I forgot I had told her that [about releasing tensions by focusing on Maisy's touch]. So I was just kind of stroking her. She said, "The whole time, I remembered wherever you touched me, I had tension, so I was concentrating on relaxing." Oops! [Laughs]. Now I try to remember what I say to people, but that worked for her.

Maisy inadvertently discovered that the power of suggestion and attention worked wonderfully with a client whose dedication to unmedicated birth had been less than enthusiastic beforehand, and where culture and language most likely played a part in the prenatal communication. Maisy was lucky to the extent that her limited ability to communicate with her client resulted in a positive outcome. In other ways, she embodied the qualities of a "good doula" elaborated by the doulas in my study.

The Good Doula

Doulas' expressed motives for doing this work are strikingly analogous to 19th century debates in the professionalization of nursing (Oakley, 1993; Reverby, 1987; Witz, 1992). Florence Nightingale envisioned nursing as a "dedicated calling more akin to a religion with little importance attached to status and reward" (Witz, 1992). The overriding priority of nursing education was concerned with the moral character of the female students, according to one nursing historian:

> The discursive function of the nurse by the champions of the Nightingale philosophy pivoted around what the nurse was, rather than what she did. Discursively, the nurse and the woman were one and the same, whilst the qualities of the good nurse were those of the good woman–sympathy, cheerfulness, self-control, unselfishness, kindness, patience, trust-worthiness, and discretion (Witz, 1992, p. 142).

Feminist sociologist Ann Oakley argues an "iron link" between nursing and womanhood is one reason why nurses continue to be in a subservient position within medicine. While some of the meaning underlying the "good woman" has changed in the past century, the doulas in my study did not challenge the link between the "good doula" and the "good woman." Lorie Nelson identifies the requirements of a good doula.

> Unconditional love. You know, willingness to work with whatever judgment comes up inside of them. I think that is the key factor in a really good doula because I believe that exhibiting caring and respect for the woman regardless of what she's going through or what she's choosing is a validating force that can change her perception of herself in a difficult situation. I think it's the most challenging thing for many us. I think it takes great physical stamina to be a doula. I think it takes a great deal of open mindedness and being willing to switch, go with the flow. I think it also takes a high level of sensitivity/perception/intuition to continually grock the energy of the room, of the parties present, and what the woman's needing. It's almost like vigilance, the way I see it, on behalf of the mother, and what she's needing, and what's going on.

Lorie's description encompasses many key aspects of the "good doula" that emerged in interviews with doulas. Unconditional love or support was a dominant theme. Being open minded and alert to the emotional needs of others was also critical. In Roberta King's definition, a good doula also needs patience and awareness that the doula's feelings and even personality will influence the laboring woman.

> Compassion, time, patience. If you as a doula are an impatient person, you're going to make the mom impatient. You need to be encouraging, you need to be somebody that can get your feelings hurt and still maintain.

Roberta also defines the good doula as someone who doesn't allow her own feelings to be hurt by the laboring woman or how the birth is unfolding. Many doulas noted how the emotional aspects of the work can cycle from the doula to the woman and back again. Emmie Ward, a doula trainer, emphasizes that good doulas are both mentally and physically strong, and explains why emotionally vulnerable women are not likely to be good doulas:

I think a good doula is one who has a very strong belief in the normalcy of birth. She's a person who's compassionate, and kind, and patient. And she has to be strong [laughter] because it is a demanding profession. And I think that's strong, mentally and physically. Because there are some people who are kind and compassionate, but they're so vulnerable emotionally that they probably wouldn't make the best doulas. A person who is rewarded by being around birth and getting families off to good starts. And, maybe a person who's invested in changing birth. I think the change agents also make good doulas. You know, the ones who are on their way to becoming midwives, or the ones who want to change birth for women so that it can be treated with the respect it deserves. I mean, I love those kinds of doulas too.

In Emmie Ward's experience as a doula trainer, she has had experience with various types of women: emotionally vulnerable ones, as well as those she describes as "change agents." She qualifies her assessment of a good doula as "maybe a person who's invested in changing births," and her final words "I mean, I love those kinds of doulas too," imply that perhaps some other trainers don't, or that these types may not be considered "good" by other doulas. Tiffany Smith continues in this vein but is much more explicit in her definition.

Good doula? Someone who's ready to jump in, respectful above all of mom's goals, decisions. A lot of doulas are anti-medical. Open and respectful of mom's choices, educated (partly through experience) about medical procedures to prevent c-section; committed to continuing education, knowing strengths and weaknesses as a person, and boundaries as a doula. We're not to be the ones advocating.

Tiffany provides the cautionary side in defining a "good doula." A nurse by training, she was also the only doula in the interviews to stress the importance of technical knowledge and education. Like Emmie, she considers it essential for a "good doula" to know "one's own strengths and weaknesses as a person and boundaries as a doula."

The "Bad" Doula

One mechanism for guarding the integrity of the "good doula" occurs by defining and identifying "bad" doulas as those who do the work for their own gratification and impose their own agenda onto the client's birth situation. Interestingly, "bad doulas" were never identified by name in interviews or in my informal discussions with doulas, and no one ever self-identified as a "bad" doula. Rae's description of the "bad" doula includes:

> She sees herself as the savior of the day who knows what's the best thing for everybody in all situations, and that's the way it's going to be. And I can think of particular people, they seem to have plenty of doula work, but I can't see them in that situation. But maybe it's a complete turnaround because they seem to need so much of a focus on themselves when I have encountered them.

Rae finds it hard to imagine how the "bad" doulas she knows could exhibit a "complete turnaround" to focus on another woman's needs during labor since, in her view, they didn't embody "good doula" demeanor in their everyday interactions with other doulas. Tiffany Smith expands her definition of the bad doula based on what she hears from obstetric clinicians, and from doulas in support group meetings.

Bad doula? Well, a complaint I hear, according to doctors, is a doula who argues with them, who interferes with medical care, and not just where mom is educated—I've heard where doulas are actively arguing with doctors about whether something is needed. Moms choose their care provider and place of birth—we have to let go of our own goals and issues. The doulas that scare me are those who say their job is to protect the mom from medical staff. And to a lesser account those who say their job is to advocate for the client. I don't think our job is to advocate for a client. I think our job is to empower clients to advocate for themselves.

Closing ranks around the desired attributes of doulas and doula practice is an important informal social mechanism for reinforcing doula norms, if basically without formal consequence. "Bad" doulas are soon identified by hospital staff complaints, and other doulas sometimes complained about having to go in and "clean up" that doula's reputation after obstetric clinicians reported negative experiences with her. In some places, members of local organizations meet regularly with obstetric nursing staff to provide in-service teaching or presentations that clarify the role and comportment of "good" doulas.

Local and national organizations usually have grievance procedures in place to address official complaints of a doula's behavior. The rogue or "bad" doula presents difficulties for all of the doulas in the local community. Because there are relatively few births in any hospital with a doula present, any one doula by extension represents all doulas. Yet there is no requirement for doulas to be a member of or certified by an organization. Indeed, in larger cities, the doulas who practice are likely to have received training and certification from any of a number of doula certifying organizations. Someone with a complaint about a particular doula may find it difficult to track down which, if any, organization the doula is affiliated with and report a grievance. Unlike a profession in the sociological sense, there are no absolute formal mechanisms to sanction or remove from practice those doulas who violate standards of practice or the code of ethics.

Gender Essentialism in Doula Practice

Perhaps the greatest contradiction of the doula role is the leveling of expertise necessary for quality labor support to one common denominator: being a kind, caring woman. The gendered dimension of this role is explicit. Although there are some men who have trained and certified as doulas, their numbers are very low. Doula trainers explicitly contrast women's and men's knowledge and behaviors at birth. As one trainer expressed this view, "We all know this intuitively, men don't. One study showed that men spend only 20% of time in close contact with women in labor. Women spend 95%. It's in our guts to know what to do."

Doula practice is explicitly considered "women's work." The term doula is itself quite gendered, coming from the Greek meaning "woman serving woman." Although the term is often reframed in the more gender-neutral designation "experienced labor companion" or "labor support person," in cases where a pronoun is called for, the feminine is used. Doulas themselves see the work as uniquely female, as Deborah Rothman notes.

Sometimes I get kind of poetic about it. It's like there's something about hearing the female voice, feeling the female hands. I've had moms who need to look at dad, but they can't stand to hear his voice. They need to hear a woman's voice, you know, and it's kind of primitive or whatever, but it's just, it's the mother voice. Not necessarily YOUR mother [laughter], but I think we need to have the support of female energy.

Doula marketing relies on this understood assumption of childbirth as a woman's affair when it emphasizes the currently unmet emotional needs of women in labor. Brochures and websites often highlight published research comparing male partners' vs. doulas' roles and activities at births (Bertsch, Nagashima-Whalen, Dykeman, Kennell, & McGrath, 1990). In explaining why so much of this research found men's activities as less than optimal, author and doula Penny Simkin writes:

Perhaps it was too much to expect of most men—to witness their loved one's pain, to nurture and encourage her in managing her pain, to act as her advocate, and to maintain perspective and confidence in a strange environment filled with busy, authoritative professional people. For most men, keeping out of the way, cooperating with the staff, and letting the staff do what they feel is best, has seemed to be the most suitable role (Simkin, 1992b, p. 1).

Men's emotional reactions to a loved one's pain are subtly characterized as not necessarily in the best interests of the laboring woman. Cooperating with medical staff is also something doulas are supposed to do; whereas a man cannot "maintain perspective and confidence" and still encourage his partner to manage her pain, the doula can. Thus, marketing literature for doula care turns the understood assumption of woman's caregiving as superior to men's at a particularly female moment—giving birth—into a careful description of an occupational niche.

Care is taken by doulas to avoid the perception that their presence at births will create a barrier between a woman and her partner, whether emotionally or physically. Doulas often sell their services to the partner as well as the pregnant woman. When asked if men could be doulas, Deborah Rothman replies:

There's another thing which doulas have, that slight bit of objectivity. That analytic mind, you know, a + b = c. That's hard to maintain when you're in love [laughs]. But men being doulas ... In general, I think that men can team with women, but I don't think you'll get the same effect if there are only men supporting a woman.

Deborah emphasizes the problem-solving capacity of the doula, made possible because she is not clouded by her emotional connection to the laboring woman. While this view inverts the stereotypical notion that women are more emotionally connected, it doesn't fully account for the separate roles of gender, partner, and emotional caregiving in the birth setting. When doulas equate their ability to be both more rational and more emotionally connected than male partners of the laboring woman, they discount the learned behavior of emotional caring and leave little space for the role of a doula in a lesbian partnership, for example. Male nurses who work in labor and delivery, as well as those men who wish to work as doulas, are also left out of this framing.

When Caring Doesn't Come Naturally

Despite appeals to the "natural" caregiving women provide other women during childbirth, one feature of doula training is an exercise to consider under what circumstances the trainee can or will not provide optimal labor support.

Here the highly charged ideological arenas of childbirth and mothering present dilemmas for doulas, whose role is to "unconditionally support the laboring woman's choices." This "values-clarification" exercise asks doulas-in-training to identify situations where their personal biases are stronger than their ability to offer unconditional support. These biases may include elective medical interventions they cannot condone, or women's choices regarding breastfeeding or circumcision.

Because they work independently, doulas have the freedom to exercise some discretion over which clients they accept. As a result, some doulas only work with women planning home births or with couples who express desire for unmedicated childbirth. Sometimes doulas seek out "difficult to care for" populations, and find a particular niche providing childbirth support for single teens, women in prison, those giving their babies up for adoption, or women undergoing drug-addiction treatment. There are a number of community-based doula programs that specifically focus on women with high social-support needs.

Doulas are often drawn to working with women who are vulnerable or have high social-support needs, especially if they have had similar experiences. Brenda Jenkins, a white mother of four in her late 30s remarked that her experience in an abusive relationship inspired her to empower other abused women during their births. She hopes the support she provides will create a foundation from which they can draw upon when/if they stand up to their abusive partners. She feels that by being a doula, she is helping victimized women at this vulnerable time in their lives as well as healing her own past.

Descriptions of doula care as a "natural talent" present a rosy view of work that can be extremely difficult and obscures the possibility that working with women in challenging circumstances may raise complex emotional reactions in doulas that they may not expect, be prepared to handle, or feel comfortable communicating to others. The birthing woman may not want a doula present, nor be grateful if one is there. A client whose care is paid for by public health funding may view her doula as yet another intrusion from the state monitoring her experience against that of the "normative" mother, represented by the doula in many respects (white, college educated, with wanted and planned pregnancies). On a physical level, the woman may exhibit behavior that is frustrating and possibly infuriating to the doula. Not all birthing mothers are "model" clients.

Empowering women in the actual circumstances of their lives and choices is not straightforward, even when individual doulas don't face dissonance between doula ideology and their own doula practice. An older, divorced white woman in her late 50s who has retired from a successful mid-level professional career in business, Rae Messenger works with many young, low-income, disenfranchised women. She acknowledges that for some of these young women:

[My being there as their doula is] not going to be important … but it's still important, I think, in the outcome of their experience of what birth was like. The idea of a woman being in that vulnerable position and at the mercy of other decisions—it's not like an auto crash, where you're half conscious, and they [medical personnel] have to do whatever they have to do. In those circumstances, most people are grateful; they couldn't have done it without help. Well, these women could have done it, and to give them that experience—a lot of young girls I see have screwed up all their lives, or have no direction or understanding of how they got that way. To them, life just happens. To give them a place where they can decide, and have someone to back them up and support them, is valuable to them whether they recognize that at the time or not.

Rae is confident that her role as a doula gives her young clients a place where they can exert agency, and she believes this is valuable to them even when they are not aware of her efforts to carve out a decision-making space for them in an otherwise overwhelming and disempowering situation.

Although some situations can be extremely unrewarding, the doula believes her job is to cope the best she can because she is there above anything else to help her client to the best of her ability. Doula Judy Dixon shares her own reaction to her first client, a woman receiving methadone treatment for drug addiction:

> [It] was really hard, she was on a really high dose, and it took her baby a whole month to detox. You know, you just want to shake her, and say, "What the fuck are you doing? Look what you've done to your baby!" But she's doing enough of that to herself. It's hard, but I think it's something we should all learn how to do [not be judgmental in words or actions]. And then yeah, maybe it would be a really sanctioned profession.

Judy's comment about doula practice being a "really sanctioned profession" addresses one tension within doula organizations and their current occupational status. The self-selection process that allows individual doulas to choose their clients means that not all doulas need to develop the skills and obtain education similar to those in other helping professions, like counseling and social work. Sometimes keeping judgment out of the birth room and helping as much as possible is not good enough, both for the doula and for the client, as Dawn Blair notes when she talks about PALS doulas' experiences with the Incarcerated Women's Project.

> There are limits to what we can provide. This is a very isolated, underserved population of women here [the County jail]. In some cases, it's been harder for them to have a doula. They need more global support. The idea

of somebody coming in and treating you kindly for a day, when you're vulnerable, and then leaving. For women who have had abandonment backgrounds, it's very hard. I've not managed to do much more than witness ...

In this fairly extreme labor support situation, the doula's clients are brought into hospitals in prison uniforms and sometimes restraints, and during labor, guards stand by, as much a continuous presence as the doula. The need for "global support": professional counseling, job training, and other social services, is beyond the scope of the doula. Despite these circumstances and the program assigning only professionally trained and experienced doulas to serve this population, Dawn notes ironically, "But our worries over connecting with our clients went away quickly. Our first referral was someone who was a doula trainer. We are us."

Debbie Oldham, a working-class white woman in her late 40s, specializes in providing doula care for extremely difficult cases, including women who are expecting to give birth to a child with a developmental disability, as well as developmentally disabled women who must relinquish their babies shortly after giving birth. She acknowledges, laughing, that this wasn't what she planned on specializing in when she trained as a doula, as they're not those "wonderful births" that are shown in the videos. But Debbie feels that she "was needed more than by the typical Mom and Dad. They need support to give that baby up." When asked why she works with such difficult cases, she tells a story about one of her clients, a young woman with the mental capacity of a six year old, who was raped in a hospital and subsequently became pregnant. Debbie says somewhat bitterly:

These women are on the lower scale of humanity. Nobody cares. "What did they do to deserve these things?" That's what the sheriff's department will ask you. [Continues in a sarcastic tone]. Well, let's see, she was lying in a bed with casts on both legs, and she said "Hi" to somebody walking down the hallway, so I guess she deserved it. So that's the exact scenario.

As the mother of a developmentally disabled child, Debbie has great empathy for the emotional and informational support women with disabilities need during labor. By creating an expert niche for herself, she gains personal and community status, if not economic remuneration, for focusing on this special population.

Emotional Costs and Rewards for Individual Doulas

Motivations—ideological and/or financial—pose tensions both within and outside the doula community. Doulas who incorporate a business rationalization into their practice are often seen in opposition to those who adopt an avowedly charitable or humanitarian role. Many business types are respected, if grudgingly, by some of the same people who express displeasure with the money-motivated doula. Doulas are unlikely to make sufficient income to support themselves financially—in my study, only a few were self-supporting from their labor doula practice. To ask why anyone would do this work without socially accepted validations such as professional status or economic benefits leaves the doula's motives open for examination, much like the physicians who incorporated holistic medicine in their practice, thereby reducing their income and peer respect considerably (Davis-Floyd & St. John, 1998). The economic benefits from doula practice, however, are meager compared to the emotional and cultural benefits that women derive from having access to births and a clearly defined, socially approved, non-medical role there.

In this context, the emotional support provided by doulas during labor is seen as one of the most fulfilling and rewarding aspects of the role.

> Though the work can be exhausting, there are unusual rewards. Doulas describe a barrage of powerful and positive emotions after a birth. They describe a unique euphoria that often lasts up to twelve hours. They feel good in a way they have not previously sensed (Klaus, Kennell, & Klaus, 1993, p. 148).

I recall from the field notes I made at my first birth as a doula:

> I came away feeling so incredibly HIGH and exhilarated. I don't know how doctors or nurses can do this, and do it so impersonally. To me, birth is sacred. There is a story surrounding each new life—connecting the story to the lives that will be responsible for this new one for some time. I am in awe of the incredible leap of faith that goes into having a baby. I felt like I passed the test. I am a doula. I can do this.

Of course, as I learned over the course of my research, most doulas do not work long shifts, day after day—unlike doctors and nurses who encounter birth as a routine aspect of institutionally located work. The doula enters hospital settings, but is not "of" them. Attending the first or even the 50th birth, is not equivalent to establishing competence as a professional practitioner. The work of obstetric physicians and nurses takes place in an entirely different set of bureaucratic constraints and professional structures (Morris, 2013).

For all doulas, but especially for the new and inexperienced, emotional responses are powerful in body and spirit. My experience demonstrates how strongly and deeply felt the first birth experiences can be for new doulas. The emotional connection to birth influences how many doulas think and feel about birth in general, and the care they provide as doulas, in particular.

The emotional connection can be both a blessing and a curse for doulas. When doulas use their bodies and voices as tools to maintain a steady demeanor in the presence of their clients, family members, and maternity clinicians, the emotional benefits are achieved with great effort, and no little cost, which belies the rhetoric of doula care being "a natural talent." Lorie Nelson describes her feelings after attending her first birth:

I felt very fulfilled. I felt exhausted. I felt emotionally raw. I was physically exhausted, but I was extremely gratified.

The embodied nature of emotional caregiving is intense during labor and birth, and it is this intensity that new parents value regarding the doula's presence. According to Rae Messenger: "They [new parents] really, really appreciate it because they really, really need it." It may be this physical embodiment of emotional rawness as well as the cultural and gendered understandings and idealizations of birth which give the doula her "high." In some circles, doulas refer to themselves as "birth junkies." When asked why she was interested in doing something that would not pay very much, a recent graduate of a doula training course awaiting her first birth, replied:

I remember Tracy [the doula trainer] saying at the training, "We are birth junkies," that's why we do this and that's why we won't make any money at it.

Framing the Birth Experience: Challenges and "Doula Doubt"

Even doulas with previous professional backgrounds in nursing or social work describe the difficulties they face to frame their clients' and their own emotional responses to the situations they see at births. They struggle to maintain both a caring stance toward the client and a professional demeanor in the presence of the medical staff. Women who have had no specialized or formal training in carework professions are unable to draw on those extra-professional resources. The function of collective support then becomes more important. Whether under the auspices of a formal organization or in informal gatherings, doulas exchange birth stories and help each other reframe birth experiences in person or in online discussion groups. The impetus for this came out of the early recognition—interestingly, by doulas with professional back-grounds and credentials (social worker, public health degrees, midwives, and nurses)—that peer support would be essential for sustaining doula practice, especially for women without prior professional training in emotional caregiving.

Despite this peer support, for some women both successes and failures with the emotional part of the job become over-ly personalized. Doulas believe a woman is in a vulnerable and emotional state during labor, but the situation of birth may carry with it emotional memories and associations for the doula because in many instances, her personal experiences of birth are precipitating factors for becoming a doula. Rae Messenger recalls her first birth as a doula, where she witnessed the husband's caring attention to his wife and was very touched by his actions. Afterward, she went home and was buoyed by excited feelings for some time. However, at four o'clock in the morning, she woke up out of a sound sleep, sobbing uncontrollably. The birth had triggered memories of the births of her own children, during which her husband was cold, distant, and controlling.

Receiving rebukes from either the client or obstetric clinicians at a birth can be devastating to a doula's sense of competency and personal worth. Examples of this can include a disrespectful attitude from a doctor or nurse, or a well-meaning critique from a midwife. At a doula retreat organized by local trainers, many women disclosed their own unexpected discovery that they felt unprepared to do the emotional support required of doulas. It was, however, a revelation for them to share their feelings with others and give it a label: "doula doubt." One self-proclaimed sufferer published her account in the local doula organization's newsletter:

Doula doubt ... may be described as a sometimes overwhelming sense of self-doubt as to one's competency in the labor room. It may or may not be accompanied by feelings of failure, maybe worthlessness, and maybe even depression. My own therapist couldn't even help me here. It was simply out of her realm (Tucker, 1999/2000).

Many factors contribute to doula vulnerability. Personal histories with birth, an insecure role within the medical hierarchy, and lack of experience are implicated in how individual doulas respond to the interactional demands placed on them to provide doula care when it doesn't come naturally.

Problematizing Caregiving within Doula Practice

Work that is defined as "caring" has been a rich source of feminist analyses that attempts to balance the humanistic underpinning of such caregiving with the economic devaluation of the work itself (Abel & Nelson, 1990; Finch & Groves, 1983; Fisher, 1990; Fisher & Tronto, 1990; Gordon, Benner, & Noddings, 1996; Uttal & Tuominen, 1999). Caregiving work embedded within reproductive contexts also poses interesting challenges for theoretical articulations of work, gender, and emotional labor since most research in this area has not examined the birth space even if it does look at mothering practice.

Doula practice provides a unique case study to examine how the gendered and emotional meanings of work are "simultaneously expected and rendered invisible." It allows us to consider how emotional labor is expressed in different forms and how its significance varies in different types of paid caregiving work (Uttal & Tuominien, 1999, p. 763). It is especially important to examine how the emotional component of intense caregiving work can be seen not merely as an example of economic exploitation and gendered essentialism, but also as a motivating factor for the work in its own right.

The doulas in my study consciously situated their work within a larger social change framework with the goal of positively affecting individual women's childbirth experiences and improving maternity care for all women (Basile, 2013; Goer, 2004). As in the case of other committed professionals, such as hospice nurses or social workers, doulas knowingly enter a field that is low paying but accorded great social value, especially among other women. At the same time, many doulas seem unaware how naturalizing labor support undermines their claim to "professional" status. Further, the competing tensions within doula organizations between increased professionalization and maintaining low barriers to entry for all women to become doulas remain unresolved.

An underlying philosophical tenet of doula practice is that every woman deserves continuous supportive care in labor. When having labor support is framed as every woman's "right," a doula who sees herself as a kind, loving, nurturing woman finds it challenging, if not impossible, to deny labor support to women who request these services at a reduced or no-cost rate. It seems crass and selfish to put a price on a "priceless service." Many newer doulas struggle with how to respond to such requests. As recently trained doulas, they are eager for clients and the experience, yet may not feel as confident charging fees equivalent to more experienced doulas. On the other side, experienced doulas feel competition from doulas who have lower fee structures and may resort to reducing their fees in order to not lose clients as well as to not feel "crass." Experienced doulas relate the hard lessons learned after granting reduced-fees to clients who then spend money on large-ticket, sometimes luxury, items (e.g., new cars, destination vacations). Midwife Gloria LeMay describes her experience in a blog post that was referenced by doulas in an online discussion about clients who wanted a "no-cost" doula:

> I have done many births in my career for free because I "felt sorry" for the couple. This is a kind of arrogance about others that usually ends in disaster. Now it seems particularly ridiculous that I did a lot of this free work when I was a struggling single parent, with two little kids who I could barely feed (LeMay, G., November 18, 2008).

In the online discussion, doulas drew comparisons with service providers, such as massage therapists, childcare workers, and even physicians and midwives who do not offer reduced fees for services. "I have to chuckle when couples are looking for a 'no-cost' doula. Were they also looking for a no-cost provider, insurance plan, hospital, and childbirth class?" (J. Batacan, personal communication, October 31, 2012).

The caregiving dimensions of doula practice, a predominantly female occupation, can be compared with the contradictions and tensions emerging in other types of care work, paid and unpaid. Sociologists Lynet Uttal and Mary Tuominen have described these contradictions and tensions "as emerging out of the clash of two value systems operating in most paid care work—the structural inequality of the labor-market devaluing of such care versus a value of emotional support and commitment in human relationships" (Uttal & Tuominen, 1999, p. 758). Doulas experience this clash of value systems when the central definition of what it means to be a competent, effective doula also includes a personal identity as a caring, nurturing woman (Uttal & Tuominen, 1999). Being a doula, for women whose sense of identity is constructed around their personal and social value as emotional caregivers, may work to their disadvantage economically although to their advantage culturally. Doulas experience the emotional consequences of the heightened contradictions around being "selfless" and "of value" at a time of socially recognized, ritualized vulnerability—childbirth. The relative low pay, long hours and emotional exhaustion pale next to "watching the universe open up."

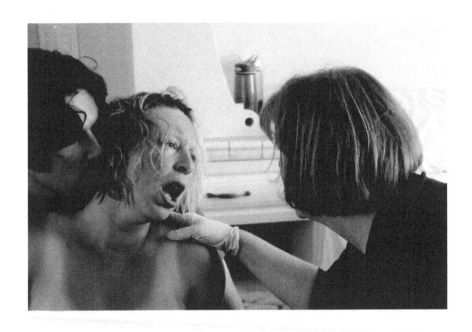

Photo 14. A doula supporting a laboring woman with breathing and vocalizations during labor, while the partner holds her.
Photo by Kyndal May.

Personal Story

"I COULDN'T HAVE DONE IT WITHOUT YOU!"
Carol Schnabel

I have been a volunteer birth doula at a small community hospital in Vermont for six years. I am middle-aged and have spent my entire adult life volunteering in a variety of capacities. Being a doula is the most rewarding of all.

Each birth is a unique event. I was so eager to become a doula, but I had no idea how much of a woman's, and, by extension her family's life is revealed in labor. It is a privilege to enter the sacred circle of birth. It is not always fun, not always easy, but always an honor. In many cases, I receive as much as I give.

My philosophy is quite simple: I am there to serve. I am there to bear witness. I am there to meet people where they are willing to be met on their journey. I leave my views and judgments outside the door. My strongest belief is that no woman should ever be alone in labor, and you can feel that you are alone, even when there are other people in the room. My mission is to do the laboring mom's bidding.

After the mother's needs, I like to focus on her partner. I believe that the birth of a baby is also the birth of a family. It is easy for a partner to be unsure how to help, to be afraid of the pain, and to feel marginalized. If I can assist in involving partners in a manner in which they are comfortable, I feel successful.

I also consider myself an extra set of hands, eyes, and ears for the nurses, midwives, and doctors. Anything I can do to help the team members ultimately helps the mother and baby. The atmosphere in the birthing room is so important.

Many women say to me after their baby's birth, "I couldn't have done it without you." It's flattering, and yet, they would have had their baby whether or not I was there. I hope I add a feeling of empowerment for the mother. She is in an alien environment, surrounded by strangers, and not feeling great. My job is to honor her feelings, give her confidence, and help create memories. Women remember the births of their babies forever. They may not remember me, but if I made this pivotal day in their lives something they are proud of, then I have done my job.

What have I learned? What have I witnessed? I have learned that too many women have histories of sexual abuse, and too many babies are born into difficult situations. Yet even in the most trying scenarios, there is joy and love at the birth of a baby. That baby will need all the support it can get in its journey through life, and that mother needs to know that there is support.

I have witnessed the grace of a hearing-impaired woman with a difficult labor who accepted each new development with dignity and joy after the birth of her daughter. Her words to me the next day, "I was looking forward to your visit," could have been my own words!

I have seen the grace of a learning-disabled woman who followed suggestions as well as or better than any other woman I have attended. I've witnessed family members and friends so involved in their own issues that labor stalls due to all the distractions.

I have seen ex-husbands, divorced parents, and many other unlikely participants come together to support a laboring woman. I have seen a family witness the birth of a daughter, sister, granddaughter, niece, and friend, during a full lunar eclipse. Including midwife, nurses, doula, and the new baby, there were seventeen people in the room at the moment of birth. It was a jubilant, respectful group. It was glorious.

People bring photos of children, pets, grandparents, gardens, and more to the birthing room. Sometimes when things get challenging, the photos are a real focus of concentration. Other times, when the labor gets difficult, the woman wants the photos out of sight.

Occasionally I am called upon to care for another child during the labor, either in the birthing room or in the waiting room. One child was only a year-and-a-half old and did not want to be without his parents. He was there for the birth of his sibling, in my arms, playing with the hat on his father's head as the baby was born. It was a blessing to have both babies right where they needed to be—in the presence of their parents.

I have seen a woman so relaxed that others around her thought she had not progressed much. In fact, she was just quietly retreating to her own private place to handle the surges. And I have been with a woman who could not relax at all. I discovered that my role was to distract her. In the midst of everything I started asking her questions about her family, her travels, and other interests. Soon the midwife and nurse realized what I was doing, and we had a gabfest. It worked!

Twice I have been at births as someone I knew was dying. Those births were a gift to me, in more ways than usual. What is better than new life and hope to restore one's equilibrium?

One woman had already discharged two of her nurses by the time I arrived at the hospital. She told me about the birth of her first child, revealing that she had tussled with the midwife. She'd also had a doula at that birth. I asked how that worked. She said, "I liked her a lot!" I knew then that I was the luckiest attendant at that birth.

Sometimes I spend a lot of time communicating with a woman in the weeks before her labor, and then she has the baby so fast that she doesn't get to call me. Still, I feel I've done my job by giving her the confidence to have the birth she desired.

The baby occasionally is born before I can get there. I try to help with the postpartum arrangements, cleanup, making sure the mother is comfortable and has food and drink. When a woman has a cesarean section, I sometimes go with her into surgery. Often I am there right up to the operation and after. There is always something I can do.

Birth stories are as varied as the people involved. I go to a birth with an open mind and with no agenda but to serve. A doula's job is so rewarding. At the end of the day, I should be the one saying, "I couldn't have done it without you!"

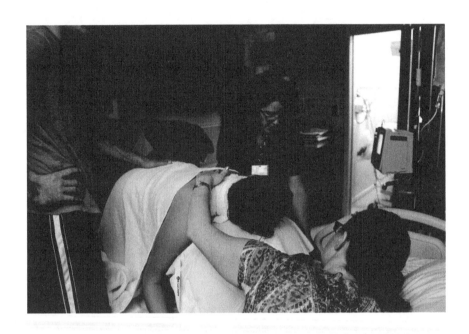

Photo 15. Doula and nurse supporting a woman in labor, using a birth ball on the hospital bed as her partner places his hand on her sacrum.
Photo by Kyndal May.

Chapter Four

Women, Doulas, and the Medical Management of Childbirth[1]

> Doulas offer a counter balance to a medical system that places an inordinate amount of value on gadgets, medicine, and machines. Helpful and often life-saving equipment need not eclipse the power of compassion.
>
> Amy Wright Glenn[2]

As discussed in Chapter One, the doula role was initially conceived to facilitate out-of-hospital birth, but it was not long before doulas sought to become a valued member of the maternity team within hospital-based births. Although doulas can and do assist at planned home or birth-center births, out-of-hospital births accounted for 1.2% of the 3,985,423 births in the United States in 2010 (MacDorman, Declercq, & Mathews, 2013). Most doulas provide labor support in the setting where most women give birth: the hospital.

In the early 1990s, when DONA International was still in the process of formation, the benefits of labor support were validated not primarily through women's experiences, but from the clinical trials described earlier that found improved outcomes of interest to the researchers (fewer cesareans, more breastfeeding, etc.). These scientific findings were accepted uncritically at first by doulas who used them to provide an

---

1 This chapter is based on the author's sociological research on the history and experiences of doulas in the United States. The methodology is described in the Appendix.

2 Glenn, Amy Wright (2013). *Birth, breath and death: Meditations on motherhood, chaplaincy and life as a doula.* Publisher: A.W. Glenn, p. 30.

insider's warrant for doulas' place as a member of the maternity care "team." Remember doula Rose Peters, comment from Chapter One:

> Anything in this OB [obstetric] or medical world has got to have a name on it. So if I could use their name to get what I needed done for the women in my area that was fine with me.

Getting what was needed done for women included "getting in the door" and articulating the scope of the labor support role. Chapter One described how early leaders in the doula movement justified and expanded their role as labor support providers in the hospital. This chapter explores more closely how doulas describe dilemmas they face and the strategies they employ to provide labor support in the highly constrained, yet dynamically interactive environment of medicalized childbirth—the hospital.

The many dilemmas doulas face are varied and generate topics for trainings, online and in-person support groups, and discussions. Chief among these dilemmas are when hospital policies or clinical practices violate or circumvent the core belief among doulas that women have the right to plan for their birth, to be active participants in their care, and to be treated with dignity and respect. As others have noted, this core belief is often at odds with the structural care models currently in place at most U.S. hospitals (Goer & Romano, 2012; Norman & Rothman, 2007).

What complicates the doula's role in this setting, then, is how to facilitate women's informed decision-making about care options and, when necessary how to mitigate gaps between the plan and the reality. How doulas do this is the subject of this chapter beginning with an examination of the context in which labor support role is carried out. This includes what women want in childbirth, and how most hospitals are set up (or not) to provide optimal, women-centered care.

What Women Want from Maternity Care Providers

Despite worsening trends in birth outcomes for both mothers and babies in the U.S., and notwithstanding critiques of mainstream obstetric care for its deficits in providing evidence-based practice and humanized care (Block, 2007; Goer & Romano, 2012), 83% of childbearing women report being largely satisfied with the care they receive at hospitals (Declercq, Sakala, Corry, Applebaum, & Herrlich, 2013). One way that doulas and maternity care advocates account for this apparent disconnect is to assume birthing women lack knowledge about what care could be like—they don't know or expect better. Another way they respond is that they attribute a "halo effect" to postpartum women, contending that the prescribed joy that surrounds a having a healthy baby takes precedence over all other feelings, especially critical ones, that a woman may have about her birth experience (Goer & Romano, 2012).

Both responses are problematic. The first assumes that all women will respond similarly to the same information and have universal needs and desires around childbirth. The second response assumes that women are what sociologist Harold Garfinkel described as "cultural dopes," uncritically accepting the overriding cultural imperative to be thankful for a healthy baby and not complain about how they were treated during birth. The plethora of birth stories shared online belies the notion that women do not recognize the complexities and, sometimes, the contradictions in their experiences.

Initially, as shown in Chapter Two, doulas and their organizations assumed that the same scientific research findings that so influenced their own advocacy would also affect their clients' beliefs and decisions about birth. Yet women are not homogenous; they differ in their beliefs and desires around birth (Gurman & Becker, 2008). Even with the same information available, women make different choices. Some pregnant woman—educated, informed, and middle class—increasingly seek humanistic care in the midst of the technological management of birth (Lake, Epstein, & Moritz, 2010; Wolf, 2001). Other pregnant women may have knowledge of alternatives but limited choices regarding birth providers or birth settings. Still others may come from cultural contexts in which, for example, a cesarean surgery, is viewed as evidence of good medical care rather than an undesired and medically unnecessary intervention (Francis, Berger, & Kim, 2008; Gurman & Becker, 2008). Finally, some women outright reject doulas and childbirth educators as authoritative critics of mainstream obstetrics care and embrace epidurals and maternal-choice cesarean as their right (Brockenbrough, 2000).

Pregnant women are bombarded by an astonishing amount of information, advice, and admonition regarding what they should do—and want—around their childbirth experiences. This often takes one of two forms. Perhaps the most ubiquitous are the personal experiences related via social media, news stories, and informal sharing among friends and family. These personal stories often assume that any one individual's choice or experience is the "right" way. The other form, coming from childbirth educators, doulas, and other maternity care advocates consists of decontextualized "universal" information and/or advice that assumes individuals have unrestricted choices regarding location or provider of care. All too often, however, this type of information ignores how healthcare practices and arrangements structure most women's experience and understanding of pregnancy and birth, limiting their knowledge of and access to a variety of options. Even when aware of their options, many women accept the passive role of patient and expect their doctors (or nurses and midwives) to navigate the medical system on their behalf (Brubaker & Dillaway, 2009).

Research that examines the beliefs and experiences of women who are located in different structural relations to the medical profession shows that women, regardless of class, want information (Lazarus, 1994; Namey & Lyerly, 2010). However, in Lazarus's research, women with low socioeconomic status exercised less choice over the selection of their doctor or prenatal clinic. With relatively little information about the medical management of childbirth, many low-income women did not feel comfortable or confident responding to questions about their preferences regarding delivery methods (Bridges, 2011; Brubaker & Dillaway, 2009; Francis, Berger, & Kim, 2008).

Sometimes, clinicians and doulas interpret women's silences during medical encounters as meaning that these patients don't care about their choices in birth settings and, as a result assume they need less support or information to make those choices. We saw in Chapter Three how doula Maisy Simmons interpreted the silence of her client, a non-English speaking woman, during their prenatal encounter as indifference to the impending birth. Lazarus concludes that middle-class women and health professionals are more able to exercise control over what they want in terms of physician care and type of birth experience compared to women with low educational levels and socioeconomic status. However, even for this relatively privileged group, she notes that what information they had "was never enough. No matter what they knew, it could not empower them within the medical system. Knowledge itself could not give them authority, nor could they know all the contingencies of the birth process or of institutional care" (Lazarus, 1994, pp. 37-38).

Information alone is not always sufficient to help women, regardless of their prior knowledge or socioeconomic status, to get the childbirth experience they desire (Wolf, 2001). Doulas thus face the challenge of describing their critique of mainstream obstetric care to women who may not share their concerns or be persuaded by their claims of worsening birth outcomes due to interventive birth practices. Doulas who are able to bridge the information gap by acting as content curators—who translate the worrisome statistics and provide warm reassurance that their presence will be valued—are the ones whose clients say afterward, "I couldn't have done it without you."

How Women Prepare for Childbirth

The contentious debates operating within childbirth practices in the U.S. maternity care system play out in a microcosm at each individual birth, in a particular location, with a varied cast of attendants. Many pregnant women and their care providers do not have a fully trusting or informed relationship regarding each other's wishes, practices, and ideas about birth other than everyone wanting a similar outcome: "a healthy baby and mother."[3] The birth plan, a one-to-two page statement of the pregnant woman's desires for and/or against interventions in birth, has long been a product of taking a childbirth education class.

Many obstetric clinicians, however, see the birth plan as an attempt to control or influence clinical decision-making by a relatively uninformed and naïve and/or ignorant consumer who is in no position to second-guess medical and clinical judgments. Because childbirth is an experience whose definition is open to dispute (pathological condition or a normal, physiological process), it opens a space for debate, questions, and alternatives and has been the major point of contention between medical and midwifery approaches; even within medical approaches such as family practice vs. obstetrics (Klein, Kaczorowski, Hall, Fraser, Liston, Eftekhary, . . .&

---

3 The presence of two "patients" during pregnancy and childbirth can complicate care when treatment for the health of the fetus may compromise the woman's health (or vice versa). Professional and personal biases or beliefs regarding which patient should be prioritized have deep religious, political, and historical contexts. Some doulas are there because of their interest in the baby; these dynamics are more fully explored in Chapter Two.

Chamberlaine, 2009). Childbirth educators have long tried to affect this space by educating women in the physiology of normal childbirth and by offering information regarding the risks and benefits of a range of interventions and procedures, all of which they believe women have the right to refuse or accept.[4]

Yet, despite promotion by childbirth educators, less than half of all pregnant women attend classes and surveys indicate a demonstrated lack of knowledge about common obstetric procedures and their risks and benefits. Data on how widespread childbirth education preparation was among birthing women prior to 2002 is not easily available, but the first Listening to Mothers national survey found that 70% of first-time mothers attended some kind of childbirth class during their pregnancies in 2000-2002. This proportion dropped to 56% in 2005, and raised slightly to 59% in 2012 (Declercq, Sakala, Corry, Applebaum, & Herrlich, 2013). Furthermore, pregnant women who take childbirth classes are more likely to be white and married and/or partnered compared to all pregnant women (Lu, Prentice, Yu, Inkelas, Lange, & Halfon, 2003).

Researchers have shown that most patients in general are woefully under-informed about medical procedures and treatment decisions (Braddock, Edwards, Hasenberg, Laidley, & Levinson, 1999), and this is true for birth as well (Declercq, Sakala, Corry, Applebaum, & Herrlich, 2013; Korst, 2012). Even with the increased amount of information available via online sources, most pregnant women are unaware of possible adverse effects of the most common procedures or treatments provided in childbirth: labor inductions, epidural analgesia, and cesarean section. Pregnant women are also ill-informed about gestational length of pregnancy and optimal gestational age at delivery. Just 21% of women who had given birth in

---

4 Except where the woman's right is disputed by the physician and adjudicated by the legal system. There have been cesarean operations performed against a woman's consent (Kolder, Gallagher, & Parsons, 1987; Purdy, 1996). See National Advocates for Pregnant Women for more recent cases.

the past year correctly identified the earliest week in pregnancy it is safe to deliver a baby when there are no complications (Declercq, Sakala, Corry, Applebaum, & Herrlich, 2013).

Whether or not childbirth education was ever truly "feminist" or "radical" is for others to debate (Edwards & Waldorf, 1984; Rothman, 1982/1991), but soon after its emergence in the 1960s and 1970s, childbirth education was incorporated into hospital educational programs, perhaps as an attempt to control the type and content of information to be less critical of typical obstetric management (Declercq, 1983).

Hospitals differ in their requirements that childbirth educators be certified by any of the major childbirth education organizations such as Lamaze International or the International Childbirth Education Association (ICEA). Some studies have confirmed the likelihood that hospital-based classes teach pregnant women and their partners to passively accept routine institutional birthing practices, while independent classes are more likely to socialize expectant parents to be critical consumers with a normal birth philosophy (Mardorossian, 2003; Monto, 1997; Morton & Hsu, 2007).

However, no matter what their underlying philosophy about the nature of birth or the rights of patients to choose or refuse treatment, childbirth classes typically provide little information about local hospital structure or policies and how these may affect the choices that presumably women are free to make (Korst, 2012; Morton & Hsu, 2007). Hospital policies differ regarding whether informed consent is required prior to each and any intervention; some hospitals require that patients sign a form authorizing the hospital to render care, including consent for any procedure deemed "medically necessary" throughout the hospital stay. The doula role was designed to address women's unmet informational and decision-making needs by having an authoritative guide present at the birth itself. The rest of this chapter will show how doulas insert what I refer to as an interactional wedge into the medical management of childbirth by opening a space between maternity care clinicians and laboring women for information exchange and informed decision-making.

What Women Encounter: Hospital Structures and Routines around Labor and Birth

Managed care, de-skilling of professional roles, and the increasing reliance on information technology have altered nurses' roles at births in the last 40 years (Chambliss, 1996; Coburn, Rappolt, Bourgeault, & Angus, 1999; Sandelowski, 2000). The increasing technological interventions of "normal" birth: induction or augmentation of labor, fetal heart monitors, IV lines, and surgical deliveries, along with the highly litigious realm within which obstetrical care is provided means that much of the nursing role is devoted to documenting data that can be used as a legal defense for the physician and the hospital (Morris, 2013). Although pregnant women expect to receive emotional, physical, and informational support from nurses, in most hospitals, obstetric nursing care is not structured to provide continuous support (Diamond, 1998; Tumblin & Simkin, 2001). Observational studies of nursing activity in labor and delivery have shown that nurses spend less than 10% of their time in emotional-support activities (Korst, Eusebio-Angeja, Chamorro, Aydin, & Gregory, 2003; McNiven, Hodnett, & O'Brien-Pallas, 1992).

Additionally, many nurses claim that their role is also to provide emotional support, and some feel threatened by doulas taking this part of their job (Hodnett, 1997; Payant, Davies, Graham, Peterson, & Clinch, 2008). While some nurses do a good job of providing both emotional and clinical care, many do not want, or are not trained, to provide hands-on emotional and physical labor support, whether for a routine labor or in the midst of a medical emergency. Many obstetricians note that their "go-to" nurses for hands-on labor support all have gray hair, implying that best providers of supportive care for physiological birth are experienced nurses.

Current nursing education and training rarely includes information and practical experience in non-pharmacological labor support techniques. As a result, most new nurses do not have the skills or knowledge around physical and emotional labor support, and few have seen unmedicated or non-interventive births (Jordan, Van Zandt, & Wright, 2008; Paterno, Van Zandt, Murphy, & Jordan, 2012). Several doulas in my study pursued nursing education and expressed surprise and dismay upon learning how little, if any, training student nurses receive in non-pharmacological labor support before their first clinical rotation in Labor and Delivery. Nearly all these doulas said they volunteered to provide a brief introduction to labor support for their fellow students, which was well received.

In addition to lack of training, other barriers to nursing provision of supportive care in labor include unit culture, competing demands, and short staffing. The Association of Women's Health, Obstetric and Neonatal Nursing (AWHONN) has identified staffing as a key contributor to patient safety, especially when high-alert medications have been administered (e.g., Pitocin for augmenting labor or magnesium sulfate for hypertension), and has issued staffing guidelines (Association of Women's Health Obstetric, and Neonatal Nurses (AWHONN), 2010). Nursing level of experience in L&D, and the nurses' belief systems about birth and labor support, are also not well documented (Davies & Hodnett, 2002; Payant, Davies, Graham, Peterson, & Clinch, 2008; Regan & Liaschenko, 2007) These factors—hospital policies and procedures, nurse-staffing ratios, the views and experiences of nurses, and how much autonomy and flexibility physicians may have—are critical in knowing whether patient's preferences, as expressed in the birth plan, may be honored.

How Doulas and Nurses See Each Other

Doulas who work in hospital settings primarily interact and align their labor support practice with one or more labor and delivery nurses who manage triage and admission of a laboring woman, oversee her care, and may or may not have a positive perception of the doula's role. Nurses may perceive the continuous presence of a doula as an implicit critique of the current system's lack of attention to, or prioritizing of woman's emotional, physical, and informational needs in the hospital setting, which in many ways, it is.

Doulas in my study complained about nurses who continually "push drugs" on their patients without regard to a woman's birth plan expressing the wish for an unmedicated birth. Given the high rates of epidural anesthesia at large hospitals, however, it is possible that nurses have seen very few successful unmedicated births, and so do not believe a woman's attempt will be successful or that her desire is authentic. Therefore, the nurse offers the medication at a time when it is convenient for her to deliver it or because she knows the anesthesiologist's schedule. There may be an economic imperative, as well, to maintain a high epidural rate in order to provide sufficient income for the anesthesia service.

In a 2010 survey of more than 525 labor and delivery nurses in Southern California, 63.3% of respondents thought women should have the "right" doula at their births, implying that not all doulas are perceived by nurses as being helpful (Perinatal Advisory Council, 2010). A small interview study of labor and delivery nurses in two hospitals in the Seattle area found that while most nurses knew about and had a generally good impression of doulas, some nurses in particular felt threatened by the doula's presence (Setubal, 2001). Nurses disliked the "bad doula"—someone with her own agenda who interferes with the medical management of the birth. This is sometimes associated with lack of experience, as one nurse explains, "less-experienced doulas come with a different idea of what labor is like. They do not have medical knowledge; they do not understand the whole process of labor and try to interfere with it" (Setubal, 2001, p. 39).

Another nurse tempers her assessment of doula contributions to labor support at the beginning of her statement, but then ends up with a global evaluation that reveals her discomfort with doulas.

> They can be nice. I don't like it when they cross over their limits, trying to tell the nurse what she should be doing. They put us in a complicated position when we do an intervention. They become uneasy as if we were causing harm to the mother. We want the safety of the baby and the mother. I don't like to have them around. I don't feel comfortable in their presence (p. 42).

Deborah Rothman, an experienced doula, acknowledged an evolution in nurses' views of doulas over time but thinks that many nurses still don't understand why women want doulas or the doula role in general.

> I think that there's certainly a professed belief in doulas all over now and I never used to be at the places that had a reputation as not liking doulas in my early years, so I got lucky that way. I still think that there's some individuals who are like, "Here's someone who wants to moan at the sunrise," or whatever, who just categorize the women who want doulas and doulas as, "You have no idea of the medical realities." Sometimes they're surprised if I seem to understand what's going on, if there's a concern.

Regardless of the knowledge base an individual doula may possess, her commitment to pregnancy and childbirth as a normal, fundamentally non-medical event, and her focus on women's emotional needs during labor, is often a direct contradiction to what her client will experience in the hospital. For many doulas, their idealized version of labor and childbirth, including a preference for few medical interventions and minimal use of pharmacological pain medication is unlikely to happen at any given birth they attend in the hospital. How labor and delivery nurses view doulas may depend on the setting or circumstance of their practice (Ballen & Fulcher, 2006; Davies & Hodnett, 2002; Deitrick & Draves, 2008; Papagni & Buckner, 2006; Paterno, Van Zandt, Murphy & Jordan, 2012; Perinatal Advisory Council, 2010; Veigaa, Lama, Gemeinhardta, Houlihanb, Fitzsimmons & Hodgson, 2011). As volunteer doula programs expand in hospitals and federal funding for community-based doula programs increases, and as more women turn to independent doulas to support them in hospital birth, research is needed to further explore nurses' and obstetricians' views of doulas (Eftekhary, Klein, & Xu, 2010).

How Doulas Provide Continuous Labor Support

The doula's role is to provide individual attention, information, and support to her client and to facilitate the same from the maternity clinicians. However, the informational and emotional support components of the doula role are not always straightforward and can sometimes come into conflict with each other. Doula Lorie Nelson reported that a doctor was "totally insulted" when her client wanted to ask questions about proposed interventions and their effect on her chances of a much-desired vaginal birth after a previous cesarean (VBAC). Lorie described her approach to this, and similar situations:

I try to talk to the client, rather than the doctor. Like the other day he [the obstetrician] walks in with the amnio hook and he goes, "OK, I'm going to rupture your bag."

And she's spread-eagled on her back, and starts trying to say, "But I have some questions," and he's sort of minimizing. So I continue to talk to her and say, "Do you understand the advantages and the drawbacks to having your bag broken?" And finally I managed to close her legs, and get the head of the bed up, which the doctor was a little disgusted with. She was able to try to have a conversation with him, you know, sitting up. We wanted to have a conversation about "Do we go on a time clock now, what is the risk of infection, can we use the bathtub, how are we limited as a result of this intervention and how might it help?" And we couldn't get a conversation going. But despite that, I felt good about my role, as frustrated as I was. I continued to help her get answers, so that when the birth was over, she got the information she needed to make the right choices for herself.

In this description of a particular birth, Lorie highlights many of the dilemmas and frustrations of the doula role. Lorie knew from her prenatal discussions that her client intensely desired a vaginal birth, and so as her doula, she reviewed possible circumstances where interventions might impact her client's chances of vaginal delivery, including artificial rupture of membranes, sometimes called "breaking the bag." One dilemma Lorie faces is that her role as an information resource may conflict with DONA International's standard of practice to not interfere with the delivery of medical care. Therefore, in the labor setting, Lorie gets around this potential conflict by reminding her client of questions to ask the doctor, rather than directly contradicting or challenging his recommendation to "rupture her bag." At the same time, Lorie physically repositions her client so that her legs were no longer spread apart and helps her client into an upright, more equal posture from which to interact with her physician.

In the midst of this activity, Lorie picked up on nonverbal cues from the doctor, which she described as "disgust." She described how the doctor minimized their attempts to discuss benefits and drawbacks of the proposed procedure: artificial-ly rupturing the amniotic membrane surrounding the fetus. Later, in the same interview, Lorie took pains to explain that she does not hold a dogmatic position on a natural approach, but she dislikes it when maternity clinicians (nurses or phy-sicians) take a uniform approach to every woman's labor and do not acknowledge the unique physical and emotional circumstances for a particular woman. She sees her role as a doula to highlight the woman's experience, so even though the interaction was frustrating, she ultimately felt good about her efforts.

Doulas sometimes find themselves in an awkward, emo-tionally charged interaction when their role to provide infor-mational support is directly opposed by an uncommunicative medical care provider or inflexible institutional policies. Dou-las also face conflicts between their desire to provide both in-formational and emotional support. A doula may know what her client is entitled to as a healthcare consumer, but drawing attention to this during the interaction with a nurse or obste-trician may be perceived as interfering with the delivery of medical care, creating conflict and in the end, contradicting the doula's role to "emotionally protect and nurture the wom-an's memory of her birth." As doulas described how they navigate these types of situations to prevent overt conflict, many repeated the phrase they heard in training workshops: "One doula in the labor room is better than several doulas in the waiting room."

Doula Strategies in Medical Encounters

As outsiders to the hospital, yet as self-professed insid-ers to labor support, doulas employ several strategies as they enact their role providing information, advocacy, and physi-cal and emotional support (Gilliland, 2011). Some strategies occur during the prenatal visit, such as becoming familiar with the client's birth plan and desires for interventions, and discussing communication and negotiation tactics should the birth plan be challenged by either the maternity clinicians or unexpected events particular to and complicating the birth. Throughout doula care, reframing constitutes a major strategy to achieve the goal of a "satisfying birth memory."

Strategies that doulas described using in the hospital setting include becoming a team player; backstage negotiations; direct confrontation, and silently witnessing depersonalizing behaviors. All these strategies are associated with both benefits and costs. The doula may be a "good" team player, but leave the impression that she is ignorant or ill-informed about birth. Requesting and using backstage time to go over various options in the situation can irritate a busy, time-strapped physician. Direct confrontation can strain the emotional atmosphere the doula is striving to control, and for DONA doulas, it is considered speaking on behalf of the client and thus outside the standards of practice. Finally, when doulas witness what they consider to be impersonal, disrespectful or dehumanizing treatment of their clients, they may be left with strong feelings of anger and frustration. In those situations, as in all births, the final strategy of "reframing the birth experience" becomes a challenging emotional task with the goal of helping the woman achieve a "positive birth memory."

Becoming a Team Player: Nurse-Doula Interactions

Most doulas report positive experiences working with physicians, nurses, and midwives in the hospital setting. Many invoke the notion of a "team player," likely influenced by Penny Simkin's article referring to doulas as the latest member of the maternity care "team," which is often included in their training packet (Simkin, 1992b). Nurses are the typically the first clinicians that doulas encounter when they arrive at the hospital to attend their clients in labor.

Whether doulas accompany the woman to the hospital and encounter the triage nurse, or arrive after the woman has been admitted, they actively assess a nurse's attitudes with regard to labor support activities in general and to doulas in particular. Deborah Rothman describes her strategy of figuring out the nurse's practice style, and adjusting to that:

Well, it's really important to get some kind of partnership set up or at least division of labor set up with the nurses. Most nurses—when there's a doula—I find that they are content with their clinical assessment-monitoring role. Or they'll be chatty and supportive that way. And there's a few that obviously love labor support, and there's always room for more labor support, you know. That way, I get to go to the bathroom, or work together, and that's really nice. But the ones that don't seem to approve of labor support seem content enough to do their clinical role, and I'm respectful of their job (Deborah Rothman).

Several doulas in my study reported positive experiences working with nurses who were happy to engage in a division of labor and leave provision of emotional support to the doulas. Naomi Olsen recalled, "One nurse said, 'I'm so glad there's a doula here, now I don't have to do this coaching thing.'" Not all nurses feel this way, and without knowing a particular nurse's proclivity, many doulas make an explicit effort to reassure nurses that their presence does not mean the nurse has been "ousted" in this area. Lorie Nelson describes her approach:

I try to ask the nurses questions that we have in a way that allows them to share their expertise. I like to develop a, "We're learning from you, what do you have to share with us," type of thing, so they don't feel sort of ousted by the doula, and that they're just like the paper-work person:

that they really have something to give to the situation.

Lorie strategically orients toward the nurse as a potential source of knowledge and information to help offset the possibility that the nurse might feel relegated to her documentation or clinical-monitoring role. Interestingly, the doula as hospital "outsider" works to ensure and reassure the insider nurse that she has a role to play or "really have something to give to the situation."

Maisy Simmons describes her philosophy and how she demonstrates to the nurses that everyone is on the same team, but with specific roles:

I consider us all a birth team, there's no, I'm on one side or another; we're all on the mom's side, basically. That's certainly the way I like to think about it. I kiss up a little bit in the beginning, I mean, not really, but I introduce myself and I usually ask the nurse what's going on, if she was there before me, and [I also ask] the mom, but it comes out from both of them while the mom's there. I say, "Oh, that sounds great," and I kind of reinforce back and forth, and it feels like a team, and I get out of her way and she does her thing, and I do mine.

Maisy initiates the interaction by asking the nurse what has occurred prior to Maisy's coming on the scene, and actively works to create a three-way dialogue between her client, the nurse, and herself. Through this approach, Maisy effectively positions herself as someone with a right to know the patient's medical history and future plan based on the nurse's current clinical assessment of the labor. She aligns herself with the plan right from the start, affirming the decisions with "Oh, that sounds great."

Although Lorie Nelson encountered resistance when she tried to create an "interactional wedge" into the communication between her client and the physician, Maisy attributes her success to her ability to establish rapport and be seen as a team player.

> I don't ever speak for the client, so negative comments I've heard from medical staff about doulas is when they get in there and start driving the birth. I'm not interested in that. This last birth I was at, the nurse was going to give her some Stadol, I think, or fentanyl, or something like a narcotic, and she had said on her birth plan that she didn't want anything to make her groggy and I know this will make you groggy. So I asked her, "Hey, do you want to ask any questions? I know you had on your birth plan you didn't want anything to make you groggy. Do you want to ask about what they're giving you?" And she asked, and they had a dialogue, so the nurse said, "Oh, I'm so glad you said something." So it was all about her [the client] and not about me. I think doulas can get a little bit high horse.

Maisy's story shows how she was able to effectively support her client's desire not to have any groggy-inducing medication by pointing out what the nurse was about to do, presumably without first informing the patient. In this way, the conversation about medication choices occurred between the nurse and the patient, not through her, the doula. Her comment about doulas getting a little high horse implies that doulas sometimes think they are responsible for making decisions or speaking on behalf of their clients, and becoming indignant if maternity care clinicians do not regard women's desires. In contrast, Maisy's story illustrates how she provides both informational support ("Do you want to ask about what they're giving you?"), and advocacy (honoring the woman's birth plan), in a way that served the client's needs and was received positively by the nurse.

Tiffany Smith, a doula and a nurse, acknowledged the potentially contradictory roles of informational and emotional support in the doula role and agreed this was an ongoing issue in both her doula and nursing practice. Tiffany's tactic is different:

> It's a balancing act, to push up to the line but not over. Always negotiation. As a nurse, one of my roles is to advocate for patients. So I use what I call my dumb nurse voice—playing stupid in a non-threatening way—non confrontational.

Tiffany's nursing experience and knowledge serves as a resource for her interactions with clinicians when she works as a doula. She told a story about a birth in which the placenta was taking a long time to come out. Tiffany noticed the doctor becoming impatient and tugging on the umbilical cord. She asked a supposedly naïve question, "Gee, how long does it take to come out?" and says, as a result "I bought the mom time, about 45 minutes, because the doctor was pulling on the cord."

Tiffany was concerned about possible hemorrhage and other postpartum complications for her client if the doctor rushed something that Tiffany knew could normally take up to an hour. She used her "dumb nurse voice" to redirect the doctor's awareness to the wide variation in "normal." In so doing, Tiffany felt that she "bought the mom time" to hold and admire her newborn before the nursing staff took the baby for institutional processing: measurements, bathing, vitamin K shots, and so on which occurs after the placenta is out. This strategy of using "classic" feminine wiles like feigned ignorance was often described by doulas when they asked a question of the nurse or doctor in front of the client in an attempt to get another viewpoint introduced. Nurses also employ these and similar strategies when faced with the power differential and differences of opinion around patient care (Chambliss, 1996; Sleutel, 2000).

Doulas describe the best nurse-doula scenario as one where both assist each other and work for the benefit of the laboring woman. Leah Lukas fondly recalled a nurse's behavior as she recounts a birth story during which the client got an epidural and fell asleep after a very long labor:

> The nicest thing for me in that birth, I was sitting next to her [the client], dozing, around 3 a.m., and a nurse came in, and put a warm blanket on me. She was a doula to me. Her intention was so sweet.

Leah's account shows that when nurses demonstrate personal, attentive care, they are viewed as acting like a doula rather than a caring nurse.

Doulas who stressed the importance of establishing a "team" approach with the nurse acknowledge that part of what the doula is there to accomplish infringes on some part of the nurse's job description: providing labor support. Doulas are aware, however, that individual nurses vary in the degree to which they embrace the hands-on labor support aspect. By making initial overtures to the nurse, the doula is able to assess the degree to which the nurse will be an ally with the doula and support the woman's desires. Doulas who perceive the nurse to be hostile to doulas or embodying a greater orientation toward official hospital policy or routine practice employ different strategies in their interactions.

Backstage Negotiations

Another strategy doulas use to counter medical information or unhelpful attitudes from clinicians occurs during their access to "backstage" time with their clients, when no clinicians are present. This strategy can utilize information obtained prenatally about the client's fears and desires for her birth and agreed-upon techniques for managing a physician's recommended intervention or change of course. Lorie Nelson describes it best.

> Well, one thing that I try to do is when the doctor's not in the room—I've encouraged my clients to say, "We'd like to think about it"—and they ask the doctor to leave, and then come back so that we have a chance to talk in privacy. What I'm finding is that the doctors have egos, and the last doctor we were with said to the client, when she started asking a few very simple questions about artificial rupture, "I've done a couple more births than you probably have. I've done about 4,000." You know, totally demeaning. And I wanted to say, "Yeah, but you haven't had your baby. You're not the one who's giving birth right now." He was totally insulted that she wanted to ask questions.

This backstage strategy can be an effective way to validate women's feelings about the medical interaction, or to sort out possible approaches to the particular situation at hand. It is also used by doulas as a practical strategy for challenging and countering medical information, and providing more "advocacy," as Tiffany Smith revealed, "As far as information/advocacy roles, what I do behind closed doors is a little bit different from what I do in front of the doctor."

Roberta King provides a concrete example of the backstage strategy to help her client achieve her goal of an unmedicated birth when the nurse actively disregarded this desire by her continued offers of pain medication.

> Another thing I do is to be that buffer in between that medical staff and mom ... because nurses will continually come in and say, "You know, you can get medication,"

and the mom says "No," and they'll come back and say "You know, you can have medication ..." So that's what I talk to the mom about [when the nurse leaves]. I don't talk to medical staff. I don't give them any decision. [I tell the client] "When she [the nurse] comes back in, just let her know that you will ask for medication, and tell her "Do not ask me again." And she told them that way. Because medical staff, that's what they do, it's nothing negative against them, they're doing their job. Since we did it that way, it didn't put pressure on them, because when you're in the midst of a pain, [laughs] if someone can tell you, "Okay, I can take you out of the pain," you know, it's difficult, it's difficult.

Roberta uses her continuous presence at her client's side to offer advice on how to respond to the nurse's continued offer of pain medication. She effectively uses the backstage time with her client to construct a response to the nurse's offer for medication that kept her, the doula, out of the interaction. Roberta didn't construe the nurses' behavior with sinister motives; rather, she saw the offer of medication as "their job" but acknowledged that this offer can be tempting to a woman in the midst of a painful contraction.

This use of backstage strategy is made possible by virtue of the doula's continuous presence at the birth. Nurses come and go, but the doula remains in the room, privy to the woman's reactions to a particular nurse and with her knowledge of the woman's goals through her prenatal contact. In cases where the backstage strategy isn't applicable or doesn't work, doulas adopt varying styles of direct communication with maternity care clinicians, whether to challenge information, suggest alternative practices, or to enlist them in helping support the woman's desires for her birth.

Unlike other patient advocacy groups which predominantly promote their positions in print and work apart from direct doctor-patient interaction, doulas enact their role in a dynamic and sometimes highly charged interactional setting in which they are the organizational outsiders (Earp, French, & Gilkey 2008). Although we've seen how doulas can orient toward nurses as outsiders to the client-doula relationship, they are nevertheless highly attuned to the nurses' institutional affiliation. As Cynthia Lynn, a doula and a nurse says, the hospital "is her place of work, it is her turf." Women who are both doulas and nurses are acutely aware of the dynamics of these two roles intersecting in the hospital.

Sometimes when doulas know a maternity care clinician is giving their client misinformation, they address the issue directly. Doula Megan Harper recalls her response when her client asked the nurse about the safety of epidurals for the baby.

The nurse answers her [client], saying, "Oh no, honey, the medicine doesn't affect the baby." Now I know this is an out and out lie. So I say, "Oh, isn't that interesting, I just read a recent study in medical journal X that says baby does get affected by medication, in this and this way. But of course, nurse Jane has been doing this for 30 years, so that is her perspective."

Megan re-enacted the sugary sweet tone of voice she used in her direct response to the nurse's claim as she told this story. She manages to provide a scientific reference for her own counter-claim, while acknowledging the nurse's extensive experience. Although her comment sounded very confrontational, since she directly contradicted the nurse, Megan continues the story by saying she was confident the nurse did not take offense or become alienated by this interaction. Megan notes "I'm a people person, if I want someone to like me, I'll go out of my way to make them and I won't stop until they do."

Sometimes doulas are not as personable or as diplomatic and are not able to smooth things over as Megan apparently did. Direct communication can be perceived as confrontation or contradiction and result in unpleasant consequences. Debbie Oldham relates an encounter that resulted in her receiving a negative evaluation from the physician who was attending her client's birth:

I had a doctor get upset with me. The client didn't want an episiotomy [a surgical cut into the perineum to widen the opening], she was adamant about that. They brought an intern in, and she picked up a syringe, fixing to give her a shot. I asked her, "I'm sorry, but what do you have in your syringe?" She said, "Oh, just a little Novocain, we're just gonna do a little episiotomy here." And I said, "If you've read her plan, you would know she didn't want that." I said, "You've got to ask her if she changed her mind." And so I asked my client, "Did you change your mind? Do you want an episiotomy?" and she said, "No, they better not cut me." So the intern told me, "Well we're gonna end up having to do it anyway [administer Novocain], if she needs stitches," and I said, "Well then, that's the time we'll do it." And she tossed the syringe back up there, and she was very angry. And I got a very bad review, because we ask them to fill out an evaluation. I think doctors have forgotten that doing that [cutting an episiotomy] without permission is surgery. Anytime you cut somebody's body, it's surgery.

Although many doula organizations specify that the doula role does not include speaking on behalf of clients, some doulas make the judgment call to do this anyway, as Debbie did. Despite receiving a negative evaluation from the physician,

Debbie expressed no regret for speaking up and preventing her client from an undesired surgical procedure. She further stated her view that physicians, by and large, do not realize the importance of getting informed consent prior to any surgical intervention.

There are other ways to directly confront maternity care clinicians without incurring their anger or frustration. Deborah Rothman serves many clients whom she describes as disempowered in general through the local doula association's contract with the county public health department. In those cases, she frequently adopts a more direct approach, especially when she perceives a gap in communication and understanding. Deborah provides an example.

There was one mom who'd had three cesareans, and she wanted a VBAC. But she wasn't even at her due date, and the baby was doing some [heart rate] decels during her monitoring, and he was transverse [lying sideways in the uterus]. And this young, what's the word, not quite arrogant, but just a kind of no-nothing intern—knowing just enough to be offensive kind of thing—was coming in and talking somewhat patronizingly to mom. And I just felt like it was really important to—because she [the intern] was kind of sugar coating things, and not quite saying, "We've decided this and there's no way you're going to get what you want." So I just felt like it was really important to say, "So, is there any chance you can move the baby? Is there any chance this can happen? Why can't we wait until she goes into labor?" Really go through each piece of why they were saying this to her because they weren't really saying it directly and who knew? She might not have even realized she was getting a cesarean until, you know [it was about to happen]. You know, the cloying smile, and trying to do that kind of questioning either with mom or encouraging her to do it so that she can see the decision-making process. But I don't think doctors could do the things that they do if they were constantly in touch with the emotional lives of themselves and their clients.

Deborah consciously interjected her own questions into this medical encounter, despite knowing this is counter to most doula organizations' Standards of Practice. Her assessment of the woman's emotional and informational needs influenced her decision to force the intern to clarify the options available by asking pointed, specific questions. She offered an account for why doctors are unable to attend to their patients' emotional lives because then they couldn't "do the things that they do." While her client did have a cesarean, Deborah felt that because of her questions, her client knew what was happening and why.

Another version of the confrontation strategy is to use backstage time to directly confront the physician or nurse, enlisting him or her as a team player in the client's birth plan. In backstage talk, with maternity care clinicians, doulas convey information about the woman's emotional needs to influence how the physician orients not only to the clinical situation, but also most critically to the woman's emotional response. Penny Simkin, doula trainer, describes how this could occur using her experience as an example:

Now, I can at times—and other experienced doulas can do this—talk directly to the physician. I've gone out with the doctor, and said "Nothing's going the way she wants it; is there anything we can do to restore some of her birth plan?" Assuming good will on the part of the physician, and the desire to make this a good experience for her. And just pointing out, "We are going down the tubes here." And I've been able to recruit them [the physicians], and the woman doesn't even know it. The doctor comes in and says, "I don't have to break your bag of waters now; did you want to wait a little bit or try walking more?" Or something like that.

In this story, treating the doctor as a potentially caring human being enables the doula to enlist him or her into the doula's understanding of the situation. This means "assuming good will on the part of the physician, and the desire to make this a good experience." Many doulas find that their particular focus on women's emotional reactions to the situation can be picked up and respected by the medical care providers. However, it is not always possible for doulas to assert their humanistic values in medical encounters.

Asserting Humanistic Values in Bureaucratic and Medical Locations

As doulas work to provide labor support that embodies their values of individual, personalized care for laboring women, they confront institutional practices that regard each birth as a routine event and a potentially teachable moment (Diamond, 1998). In these cases, doulas work to convey the uniqueness and particularity of this experience both to their client and to the obstetric clinicians. Maisy Simmons describes a dilemma she faced while coaching a client through pushing during the second stage of labor.

> A nurse was there, training another nurse, and was telling her, "I always prepare the baby station as if I'm preparing for a resuscitation." [My client is] pushing and she's thinking about her baby being dead because this nurse is talking about resuscitating a baby up here, and [I was] thinking about trying to pull her back out—because she heard that—she went through a little crisis because of it, and you know … and so it's hard.

The presence of a routine teaching moment makes the interactional accomplishment of emotional support and physical coaching during the pushing phase more difficult for the doula. In monitoring the environment for practices or statements that might affect her client's emotional state and confidence, Maisy had to reassure her client that the nurse's statements were part of an institutional routine, not particular to her baby. Lorie Nelson echoes this critique of nurses' orientations toward birth.

What's hard for me is the factory mentality of many of the nurses. [INT: How does that present itself to you?] Well often, the nurse who's coming on the next shift comes in the room, and she hasn't gotten the report yet, so she walks in and with no history that we've been laboring for 60 hours, she'll just say, "Oh, I see you have the Pitocin [artificial hormone used to stimulate labor] going, you should be going any minute now." Well guess what, we've been at 4 centimeters for 30 hours. I don't think we'll be going any minute now, you know what I mean? So they're not fully informed before they'll come on. That's really challenging for me.

Not only nurses, but doctors can be insensitive to the particular needs of the individual woman, as Deborah Rothman recalls:

It's very hard when a doctor seems to be disrespectful or not knowing what's going on—just sort of talking by rote. Like I had this one client where oh, she really wanted a VBAC. She'd had two cesareans, and she dilated really smoothly, you know, normal progress, and she pushed for two hours and just couldn't make any progress, and then got an epidural to see if that would relax things and let the baby come through. And the doctor came back after a couple of hours and he said, "Well, your cervix hasn't really changed in these past few hours," and it's like, what cervix? You know, she's pushing, she's in the second stage now, and he—but I couldn't say that. So once the doctor's going around these waters where you're getting ticked off, it's really hard to know what your role should be because you don't want to create antagonism. You don't want to create a little war where mom is sort of like, "Huh?" Because that will not really help her do the task at hand.

As Deborah notes, when maternity clinicians make comments that do not reflect the particular circumstances of the woman's labor, doulas may become frustrated and angry. Doulas often interpret the clinician's comments as unhelpful and disrespectful, as well as uninformed about women's true desires or needs. When obstetric clinicians make insensitive remarks, doulas then have to modulate and control their responses, as Roberta King describes:

Now there was one time when the doctor looked at this lady, when he looked at her, he said, "Natural redhead," and I found that very crude. He came and he was talking to someone else and he said, "We got a red head here." I just looked at him and I just stared at him. [INT: Because he wasn't looking at the hair on her head]. No, right. Right. What I did was talk to the mom, I really don't know whether she heard them or if she picked up what they were talking about. I was upset about that. Did I say anything to him? No, because I know that when you're in somebody's hands, medically speaking, before anything happens is not the time to upset anybody.

Roberta wasn't sure if her client heard the physician's insulting remark, but she realized it was not something to make an issue of at the time. Despite witnessing depersonalizing behavior of this type, doulas like Roberta feel that making "a little war" or "upsetting anybody" will not serve their client's needs. In this way, they are similar to nurses who may also witness unprofessional or degrading treatment. Yet in contrast to nurses, doulas' independence from medical hierarchies and hospital employment puts them in a unique and potentially powerful situation. In online forums and discussion groups, doulas describe and share their experiences with particular doctors or nurses at specific hospitals. They write formal letters of complaint to hospital administrators. They form local associations or advocacy groups to inform women, and each other, about preferred providers and practices, as well as those to avoid. Doulas and other birth workers ask each other for recommendations for maternity providers who are VBAC-friendly, or who are known to support women's desires for physiological birth.

Doulas in my study served a range of clients, including incarcerated women and developmentally disabled women giving birth to infants they would surrender to Social Services. They served a large population of non-English speaking recent immigrants, as well as women receiving medical assistance. Doulas also served women from more privileged economic backgrounds. The differential care received by poor maternity patients is well documented (Amnesty International, 2010; Bridges, 2011; Strong, 2000). Community-based doula programs, which train doulas who match their clients in terms of race/ethnicity, socioeconomic status, and other characteristics, are emerging to take advantage of the provisions in the Affordable Care Act to provide labor support under Medicaid programs.

Doulas are a window into institutional routines and practices around birth for women of both low and high socioeconomic status. The phenomenon of disrespect and abuse that occurs in facility-based childbirth is an issue receiving attention globally (Bowser & Hill, 2010), but has not been investigated fully in the U.S. context. Doulas, as independent witnesses to facility-based childbirth in the United States, provide an important and little-known perspective on this issue.

Medical Maltreatment of Birthing Women

The extreme cases of medical maltreatment of women giving birth are a case in point. Doulas sometimes witness what they consider institutionally sanctioned rape of American women at birth, and speak of helping women endure mistreatment while feeling helpless to intervene. Two ethnographies of maternity care from the 1970s highlighted the routine physical and ideological degradation of women's bodies as part of dehumanizing birth protocols (Scully, 1980; Shaw, 1974). More recent nursing and medical memoirs about current maternity care paint a less grim picture, but still point to abuses and institutional practices that are dehumanizing at best, and coercive or neglectful at worst (Diamond, 1998; Harrison, 1982; Kitzinger, 2006).

While egregious cases of obstetric maltreatment do not occur frequently in doulas' stories, more common are cases in which a woman's desire for an unmedicated birth is not respected, or when interventions are proposed without allowing for a full discussion of risks and benefits. These are often accompanied by what doulas call "the dead baby card": when clinicians implicitly or explicitly convey the idea that a woman's noncompliance is likely to result in harm to the baby. Some of these cases involve women with a history of sexual abuse whose past experiences emerge as salient during labor, birth, and breastfeeding.

Other incidents described by doulas involve physicians who exercise and abuse their position of trust and power over women in vulnerable circumstances. Doulas confess feeling little recourse at the time they witness their client's unnecessary pain and suffering. Jodi Park relates two particularly troubling incidents she observed while working as a hospital-based childbirth educator.

[One was a] horrible doctor, I wanted to blow up his car afterwards. It was at the hospital where I work as childbirth educator, and I was observing a birth. This doctor was sewing up a woman without anesthesia. She spoke no English, and the nurse had to leave the room because she couldn't take it. All I could do was hold her hand, and watch this man abuse this woman. It was horrible. There was no excuse for it. Another time, this doctor was standing in the corner with his arms crossed. The woman was pushing, and the doctor said, "I won't deliver that baby unless you put your legs in the stirrups." I was helpless.

Stacey Kinney says that out of the 70 or so births she's attended as a doula, there has only been one doctor that she would refuse to work with again. She was working with a Chinese client who chose this particular doctor because he spoke her dialect.

That was her only criteria, so that if she needed to speak her dialect he would understand, but she spoke English the whole time, so it really didn't matter. She was 38 years old, and when the doctor came in—before she was ready to start pushing—he said, "I'm going to cut an episiotomy now." She said, "I don't want one," and he said, "You're almost 40 years old, and you're Chinese, and it's your first baby. It's impossible for it to come out without an episiotomy." And she said to him, "I'll take my chances." I could have kissed her on the lips when she said that. I was so proud of her because that's hard, for her culture, to speak up to a doctor. It was hard for her, and she did it. He tore his gloves off and threw them on the floor and said to the nurse, "When she's ready for her episiotomy, you can call me," and he left the room. She started to push, and the nurse called him and he didn't come, and when the baby's head was out, she called him and he didn't come. And he didn't come back until she was nursing her baby. [INT: What, who caught ... ?] The nurse caught the baby, laid the baby on the mom's stomach, caught the placenta, and the doctor came in. The placenta was out, the cord was tied off and the baby was fine. I told her she was so lucky he wasn't there. It was a great delivery—the baby came fast, but the nurse did a great job. The doctor came in, and said to the nurse, "You did this?" and I looked at him, and I looked at my client, and I said, "No, actually she did this—all the nurse did was catch the baby because it came out." So then he said, "You tore, you have a second-degree tear," and I said, "Isn't an episiotomy considered a second-degree cut?" and he said, "Yes, but it's straight," [INT: Did he stitch her up?] Yes, he stitched her up, but anyway the reason I wouldn't work with him was afterwards he took some hemostats, and some four by fours [cotton gauze], and clipped the four by fours together, and he started reaming her out [manually evacuating her uterus] to make sure there were no blood clots. This is a woman who had no epidural, no pain medication, she was screaming, she was trying to climb off the bed. He was doing it like the Roto Rooter man. It was horrible. I was crying, she was crying, the nurse had tears in her eyes. Afterwards, I talked to one of the other nurses, and I said "I just saw the most horrendous thing," and she said "'Oh, the thing with the four by fours?" and I said, "Does he do that with all of his clients?" and she said, "Oh, the butcher, yeah, he loves that." The nurses call him "the butcher." [INT: Oh my god!] Yeah, so it wasn't just me. This man doesn't deserve to be working with women at all. He is a horrible person and if anyone tells me that he is their doctor, I will do everything in my power to get them to change.

This doctor's use of sterile 4x4 gauze cotton pads to physically wipe out the woman's uterus and vagina has no clinical justification; it represents an outmoded standard of practice.

Yet during this extreme and medically unnecessary procedure, Stacey could only stand by and witness. Later, upon learning that his behavior was standard and known to all the nurses, Stacey vowed to alert any future client and warn them away from him.

Bearing witness to dehumanizing treatment of birthing women takes its toll on doulas. Carrie Monroe, who has worked as a birth doula and doula trainer for more than ten years acknowledges "If I didn't do so many home births, I don't think I could do this work." And Betty Wagner, who has been to a few midwife-attended births but primarily works with women giving birth at hospitals with obstetricians, rages "I get so sick of these doctors, just butchering women. And then they act like gods about it, expecting thanks."

Doula practice opens a window into obstetric maltreatment of women that allows non-medically trained women to witness and give voice to these practices they know are inappropriate. Family members, friends, and birthing women are often unaware that these practices are not necessary. Nurses also witness such practices, but are bound by institutional hierarchies and local cultures that affect how likely they are to report such maltreatment given their status as hospital employees with less professional power than physicians (Chambliss, 1996; Diamond, 1998; Sleutel, 2000). Nurse-researcher Audrey Lyndon and her colleagues found that many obstetric nurses do not speak up when they witness any practice or action likely to cause the patient harm (Lyndon, Sexton, Simpson, Rosenstein, Lee, & Wachter, 2011). One reason among many cited by Lyndon for why nurses do not speak up is the fear of jeopardizing long-standing work relationships.

In contrast, doulas who work at different hospitals and do not feel allegiance to any hospital or its maternity clinicians can spread the word about particular doctors' practices through their personal networks (including online) and thus to potential clients, as Stacey Kinney plans to do. However, doulas in smaller communities, or those who work in hospital-based programs, face similar concerns as do nurses about making formal complaints about such maltreatment, fearing reprisals regarding their reputation and ability to continue to work as doulas.

In the 1960s, the cultural taboo around mentioning the words breasts or breastfeeding, was a significant barrier to women who wanted to learn how to nurse their newborns (Raphael, 1973). Today, doulas have revealed another taboo when they bear witness to birth as sexual violence against women as in the cases mentioned above, and through their work with clients whose labor and birth trigger memories of past sexual abuse (Simkin & Klaus, 2004; Sperlich & Seng, 2008). In response, some doulas seek more information through specialized trainings on how to support childbearing women with abuse histories.

Reframing the Birth Experience

Doulas see and hear multiple perspectives on the births they attend. In addition to the evolving doula discourses on birth, they often are privy to backstage talk by obstetric clinicians as well as private exchanges within the family. Doulas may act as a communication bridge between the couple and their maternity care providers. By virtue of witnessing events at the birth and listening to multiple perspectives, doulas are in the unique position of offering a reframing of events. Doulas can also fill in the gaps in the woman's later memory of the birth and insert a heroic story about the woman's achievement. Doulas reframe the birth experience as an occasion for validating women's reproductive agency as they become mothers.

Doulas accompany laboring women on a journey through relatively unknown, uncharted terrain. Doulas, as Pam England has said, are like sherpas who mediate a great cosmic experience for the casual or new observer who doesn't know how to frame or see the experience in its fullest sense. Doulas see emotional regularities in the birth space and setting that "pregnant tourists" do not since they only pass through the space once or twice. Doulas, like sherpas, have power that comes from knowing the landscape, understanding their mediating role, and, most critically, exercising their allegiance to the woman rather than the hospital or the physician.

Doulas frame the experience for birthing women and their partners, especially around expectations for how long it might take, as Maisy does:

This husband had it in his mind—he'd watched TV births, you know—two hours into it, after the induction, he was just shocked they didn't have a baby yet. So I had to say, "Yeah, this can really take a while, are you doing okay?" Sometimes give them attention too, to make sure they get nurtured. It's so much about the moms, you know, but the dad's got to feel good and competent.

Doula and doula trainer Emmie Ward notes she often provides couples with a frame for how they handle labor without her, explaining why she doesn't go to the couple's home for labor support but instead meets them at the hospital.

I think it's rather empowering for them to see that they are strong, and that they can conduct themselves in early labor by themselves with a little encouragement by phone. And I think they're pleased to be able to look back and say, "You know, we handled labor pretty well until we were at three centimeters," or whatever it is. That they were able to do that at home, on their own.

During the postpartum visit, the framing of the birth can help fill in gaps in couples' memories about how involved the physician was, as Emmie Ward explains:

I consider the postpartum visit a social visit, and I want to hear the mother tell me her story about birth. I want to focus on that and I find she's really willing, and maybe even eager to tell me about what she remembers about the birth. And then often she'll have questions. She can't figure out why things happened, or that kind of thing, so I fill in the spaces as I remember them from her birth. Also I give my interpretation of overall how the birth unfolded—maybe some things that she wasn't aware of that are just interesting to her. Sometimes people don't think that the doctor was at all involved. And they may have feelings that they were neglected. And so I often will say, "You know, every couple [of] hours the nurse came in and encouraged you," or "She came in more often, but after a couple [of] hours, she would go call your doctor and tell your doctor how you were doing." And sometimes, they don't know that. They think that this doctor wasn't doing anything for them until the very last minute, when he came in to catch the baby. Yeah, so I like them to know that the whole team was there for them. Keeping a watchful eye on them. That maybe she was doing so well that the doctor didn't have a need to come in, you know, that kind of thing … and there are other things that she might not have known about. I think one of the reasons to do that follow-up visit is to clarify in her mind things that are questions. But especially to get at her interpretation of how the birth went and to see overall, does she feel pretty good about how she handled her labor. What's the feeling she's left with, the memory she's left with after the birth?

As we've seen, doulas may fall on any point along the natural childbirth-midwifery-medical continuum when it comes to their personal preferences and beliefs regarding interventions, especially non-medically indicated ones. It is easier for some doulas than others to accept and be nonjudgmental of a woman's choices regarding her birth as best for her. For those who stand on the far edge of this continuum, strongly believing in few to no interventions and no pain medications, a doula may represent a compromise, even a co-optation of these ideals, which helps to explain why some homebirth midwifery advocates question whether "doulas are making birth better for women or making women feel better about their births" (Norman & Rothman, 2007, p. 262).

Doulas across the spectrum from newly trained to long-time trainers acknowledge the possibility that they help women accept a non-optimal experience in the hospital. Doulas also carefully redefine the "ideal birth" from what happens in terms of interventions to how the woman feels about what happens at the birth. They also note that many women do not have a choice to have midwives or non-hospital births, and these larger structural constraints are not something doulas can easily change. In a dialogue with Kris Turner about how she reconciles these contradictions in her practice and in training workshops, she reframes this critique by focusing on women's agency within the constrained environment.

[INT: Are doulas co-opting their "ideals" by helping the woman see this birth, with these interventions, as this heroic accomplishment? On the other hand, what's wrong with telling her she's accomplished something; that she did a great job and there are people who are proud of her?] You're right, no matter what the circumstances. It doesn't necessarily seem to me to be a contradiction to say to somebody—because I see it—it's not like I'm making it up. It's not like I'm thinking I'm going to tell her how good this is and all I see is the machinery or something. I really do see it in women when I'm with them during labor. I really see something phenomenal that happens in them. And anytime I think we have the opportunity to witness that, we can amplify it by mirroring it back. It's not like we're generating it, or creating it for them, it's just that we see it, and we can reflect it back to them.

Kris points to a key way in which doulas authentically reframe the birth—they acknowledge the technology, the interventions, the maltreatment, but they also highlight the woman's agency, effort, and subjective sense of accomplishment. The doula reframes her own vision so that she sees beyond the technology and the medicalized setting and personnel that may seem to dominate the labor and birth experience. She sees something "phenomenal" that happens in women, regardless of the physical circumstances surrounding the birth.

When things haven't gone as the client desired and the doula has been unable to employ any effective strategies at a particular intervention point, she waits for the postpartum meeting to talk about what happened. Deborah Rothman describes her approach after a potentially disappointing birth experience for the doula or her client:

So depending how tired I am or whatever, you know, I'll try to think of something to say, or talk to mom and try to get her to say something, but sometimes you just sort of end up accept—you know, biting your tongue, and being ready to again talk with mom about it later. In a way that will both expand her thinking about it, and let it be something she can live with.

Deborah's comment points to the limits of doula reframing, whether stemming from her own exhaustion after a long labor or an inability to think of something to say. She starts to say, "you sort of end up accepting," but cuts off the word accepting in mid-sentence in favor of "biting your tongue." She points to the dynamic possibility of returning to the problematic situation in the postpartum visit when she might be better able to help the woman understand what happened and why, and provide resources to her for ongoing recovery and sense-making about the birth.

In reframing the birth experience, then, doulas work to highlight the arbitrary, chance elements for why the birth happened the way it did. Doulas "reframe" the woman's experience—in part because they really believe that every woman can birth a baby and be a warrior princess while doing so. Doulas acknowledge they do not independently raise their issues of concern—events from the birth that in their minds were inappropriate or misguided—if the woman doesn't refer to them as a point of concern. However, if a woman does bring up an issue, the doula does not deny or minimize the woman's emotional reaction but instead validates the complex, and often contradictory, feelings that she may have about her birth experience. In the woman's larger social network, negative feelings are often invalidated or discounted when family or friends ask a still grieving new mother "What does it matter if you had a cesarean? You had a healthy baby, didn't you?"

Doulas as Experts within the Medical Management of Birth

Doulas see themselves as complementary to each type of maternity care provider—nurse, midwife, or physician. Because they have no medical training or credential, they cannot position themselves as superior to or as a replacement for these obstetric clinicians. Yet in their claims to understand and respond to women's emotional support needs in labor, doulas and their organizations occupy an uneasy position on the role of and claim to expert knowledge. The boundaries of expertise blur when doulas theorize and attempt to influence the complex interaction between clinical practice, women's emotions, and the physiology of labor (Hunter & Deery, 2008).

Doulas, with their close attention to birthing women's emotions as well as their physical comfort in labor are the most likely experts in this domain. The physical and emotional connection between doulas and their clients may facilitate a deeper relationship. Birthing women trust their doula, sometimes more so than their obstetrician, and feel doulas have their best interest at heart. The doula has been to the couples' home; she has been with them continuously since they called her during labor, and she has placed them and their needs at the center of her care. The stories included in this volume attest to the emotional impact of the doula's role at women's birth. Yet despite the strength of the emotional connection doulas may have with their clients, their claims to obstetric science and clinical practice are less strong and more likely to be challenged by obstetric physicians and nurses.

Doulas claim familiarity with the latest scientific research and use this knowledge to support their assertions that many mainstream obstetric physicians do not practice evidence-based medicine (Goer & Romano, 2012). Yet, this familiarity and critique is easily ignored or discounted by professional organizations representing obstetric clinicians. Until mainstream professional groups recognize, define, and adopt a "problem" within maternity care, whether it is availability of VBAC or readiness of hospitals to manage an obstetric emergency, doulas and other normal birth or midwifery advocates are largely on the sidelines. Their circle of influence extends to each other and the women they serve.

Consider the example of elective deliveries (inductions and scheduled cesareans) before 39 completed weeks' gestation. Tracking these elective deliveries with the goal of reducing them to below 5% is now a national quality initiative, after the Joint Commission included this measure it its revised 2010 perinatal core measure set. ACOG's practice bulletin on the inadvisability of elective deliveries prior to 39 weeks' gestation has not changed since its publication over 30 years ago, and the clinical evidence of maternal and neonatal health risks of this practice is considerable (Main, Oshiro, Chagolla, Bingham, Dang-Kilduff, & Kowalewski, 2010; Oshiro, Henry, Wilson, Branch, & Varner, 2009). Indeed, from 1990 to 2006, there was a rise in late preterm births (those occurring between 36 and 38 weeks completed gestation), and the average gestational age at birth in the United States decreased by a full week during this time period (Fleischman, 2011).

In 2010, as a response to the increased health risks to babies born early, The March of Dimes launched a multi-state quality improvement initiative to help hospitals reduce rates of early elective deliveries, largely through implementation of a toolkit supported by the California Department of Public Health: *Elimination of Non-medically Indicated (Elective) Deliveries Before 39 Weeks Gestational Age* (Main, Oshiro, Chagolla, Bingham, Dang-Kilduff, & Kowalewski, 2010). Upon posting the link to a news story on this project to an online newsgroup, Jeanne Batacan, a local doula/childbirth educator, highlighted this quote from nurse expert Debra Bingham, an author of the Toolkit and vice president of the Association of Women's Health, Obstetric, & Neonatal Nurses in Washington, D.C.: "I've had experience with women who clearly didn't understand the risks of an elective induction, but it's also fair to say that there are a lot of doctors, nurses, and childbirth educators who aren't aware of the risks" (Debra Bingham, quoted in Johnson, 2010).

In response to the nurse expert's quote, Jeanne, the childbirth educator notes:

> I can understand woman not understanding the risks— they are not being allowed informed consent. I cannot understand "a lot of doctors and nurses" not knowing the risks. That is unacceptable, as it is their job and responsibility to know. As a childbirth educator (ICEA), I've known the risk for many years. So, it is unacceptable for a certified childbirth educator not to know the risks either.

The article points out "the entire bell curve has shifted. Now, more babies are born at 39 weeks than at full term." But fails to mention the other important issue—that the average primip gestation lasts about five days longer than average. When this is factored in, a primip being induced is at even more risk. (Jeanne Batacan, SouthBayBirthCircle@yahoogroups.com, December 26, 2010).

Jeanne's view is that since she, as a licensed childbirth educator has known of the risks for several years, then it follows that labor nurses and obstetricians should know about the risks of early elective delivery. Her comment clearly implicates clinical practice as a more likely factor in the shifting of gestational age than women's preference. She also refers to additional scientific information, though without providing a source, implying the average gestation among primiparous women (primips, or first-time pregnant) is also an important factor in babies being born too early.

Doulas, as noted earlier, are avid information seekers and critical consumers of scientific research on childbirth practices and outcomes. Like Jeanne, they are frustrated by the apparent ignorance of maternity clinicians on issues that seem clear-cut in the medical literature. In their promotion of normal, physiological birth, doulas draw on research from many fields whereas obstetric nurses and physicians are more likely to rely on their professional associations (AWHONN and ACOG, respectively) and their affiliated journals for relevant information. Doulas also attend conferences that feature sessions promoting the evidence behind normal, physiological childbirth from multiple disciplines, whereas the majority of obstetric conferences (nursing and physician) are focused on clinical pathologies or emergencies and medico-legal issues.

It is not surprising, therefore, that there are disconnects between what doulas and obstetric clinicians view as the most pressing problems in maternity care. What is surprising is that there hasn't been more conflict between these groups.

While there have been physician-group practices that have decided they will no longer work with particular doulas unless they have been "pre-approved," widespread evidence of this is difficult to determine.

Conflicts have emerged more frequently within in the microcosm of individual births, and stories of these conflicts appear in online or in-person doula support groups. These stories focus on nurses and doctors who complain about the "bad" doula, her confrontational style, and her agenda for a natural birth. The typical critique levied at these "bad" doulas is their outspokenness, their distrust of the obstetric clinicians, and their stated need to "protect" their client against non-medically indicated interventions. The truly "bad" doulas may be sanctioned as a result of formal grievance procedures, but these are typically handled as confidential matters within a doula organization, if applicable. Yet many doulas don't belong to formal organizations, and as an unlicensed occupation, doulas are not governed by licensing boards or regulatory agencies. Thus, doulas remain self-proclaimed experts in the arena of normal birth and arbiters of good obstetric practice. Their interpretation of the clinical literature supports their argument that non-evidence-based care is linked to poor maternal and neonatal outcomes. Their advocacy for midwifery care and evidence-based birth practice comes from their sincere and passionate desire for improvement in maternity care.

The Doula's Role in Quality Improvement in Maternity Care

What role can doulas play in ongoing quality improvement in maternity care? Childbirth, as a physiologic process, highlights the boundaries represented by health and illness, by pathology and normality. Are obstetricians right to claim authority in normal pregnancies and childbirth? Who can define normal? When does normal become not normal? Despite a key interest and belief in normal birth, doulas are not clinicians and do not have the ability to define a particular birth's departure from normal within the clinical setting. Doulas advocate for their clients' desires to have a normal birth, and believe that the use of certain procedures or medications at the outset of labor (IV fluids, Pitocin, epidurals, confinement to bed) may contribute to the need for yet more procedures, leading to what doulas see as unnecessary cesarean sections and subsequent health issues for women.

Doulas assess the dynamic interactional contingencies within a particular labor scenario, and weigh the consequences of their actions given the particular needs of the client and the relationships the doula has (or has not) cultivated with the attending clinicians. It is a challenging task, especially when doulas see events unfolding that are likely to result in unfavorable or undesirable birth outcomes for their clients. Despite the doula's goal to empower women and help ensure a satisfying birth experience, there are limits to what the doula can do to intervene in the clinical course of care, as doula trainer and author Penny Simkin thoughtfully observes:

> Is it empowering for a woman, a laboring woman, to have someone else speaking for her? So there's every reason in the world, as I see it, for the doula to be there to facilitate the woman's speaking for herself, to help her recognize—because this is not always clear—that her birth plan or her ultimate goals are being compromised by this particular course of action. So keeping her and her partner informed, and allowing them to speak for themselves—if they wish to—because one of the things that has shaken me a bit is that sometimes I care more than they do (P. Simkin, personal communication, February 15, 2000).

Doulas do indeed care. By placing that care at the center of their role, doulas highlight not only the importance of birth, but also raise the critical question of whose right and responsibility is it to care about how a woman's birth unfolds.

Doulas occupy the large interactional space vacated by many (but not all) nurses and childbirth educators who have abandoned childbirth advocacy as a part of their role. How interactions around decision-making are negotiated in real time, whether in prenatal negotiations around scheduled inductions or cesareans, or in the context of ongoing labor management in the hospital have been a critical gap in the research literature (Morton, 2009). In the worsening climate of maternal and neonatal outcomes and the new interest in bringing quality improvement initiatives into maternity care, the time is ripe for a better understanding of the processes by which these decisions are made. Doula practice highlights the changing relationship between healthcare practitioner and patient with regard to informed consent and shared decision-making. By inserting an interactional wedge into doctor-patient or nurse-patient communication, doula practice demonstrates the critical importance of clear communication and information exchange in order for women to make informed decisions prenatally and in the course of labor.

Although the doula is enjoined by her scope of practice and code of ethics to be completely supportive of her client's choices regarding her birth, the doula is not, and, I argue, cannot be neutral in this space. She negotiates the immediacy of labor and birth in a medical environment in which she may or may not have prior formal training in emotion work, obstetric nursing, or midwifery. She is there to assert the primacy of continuous support—the therapeutic value of a calm voice and a reassuring touch. Her role is additionally charged with the competing ideologies surrounding birth held by others in the room and the interactional necessity of having to, in the moment, provide attention that is perceived as authentically produced and demonstrated.

The doula is accountable to the client for her demonstrable presentation of emotion. She is accountable to obstetric clinicians as being competent in their discourse and respectful of their authority in a domain she has no professional claim to (medical knowledge and responsibility). Finally, she is accountable to the wider community of doulas in which she operates. Doulas who seek professional recognition in communities or hospitals that may not be openly receptive to their role at births are sensitive to how any particular doulas actions will be perceived. An activist doula, or "bad" doula, will impact more than just her own livelihood. The future of the doula role rests in part on how individual women working as doulas manage the ongoing demands and contradictions of doula practice.

The growing awareness of how health and emotions intersect provides another context for considering the impact of doula practice (James & Gabe, 1996). Doulas place women's emotional needs at the center of their birth experience, arguing that these needs have been neglected in medicalized childbirth. Opening up emotional issues within medical encounters highlights the schism between professional expertise and the women's subjective experience of childbirth.

Finally, doula practice highlights the increasingly dynamic social organization of work within healthcare settings. Patient safety and quality improvement advocates require that healthcare providers adapt to a team management model and move away from an autocratic, physician-dominated care model. This presents new ethical dilemmas for all participants, as sociologist Dan Chambliss has noted in his research on ethical issues facing nurses:

> When power relationships are stable and unchallenged, there will be few ethical crises; the answers are routinized, the decisions are made by clear authorities, and subordinates do their jobs, and keep their mouths and minds shut. But when the authorities become challengeable, when new constituencies come into being, when new occupa-

tional groups begin to define and defend their own turf, then the moral agendas of these various groups come into conflict (Chambliss, 1996, p. 99).

As much as doulas strive to be the "latest addition to the maternity care team," their limited presence at U.S. births has not yet generated a strong enough moral agenda to stand alongside that of obstetricians, maternity nurses, and hospitals. Doulas' claims to expert knowledge, and to the evidence supporting their impassioned critique of obstetric practice and outcomes, are not yet fully recognized by mainstream obstetric professional organizations. Doulas struggle to sustain their practices, as individuals and in their multiple organizations, and have, as yet, been less effective in advocating for humanistic care during childbirth within a medical and institutional framework that does not put women's emotional needs, or perhaps even their emotional health, at the center.

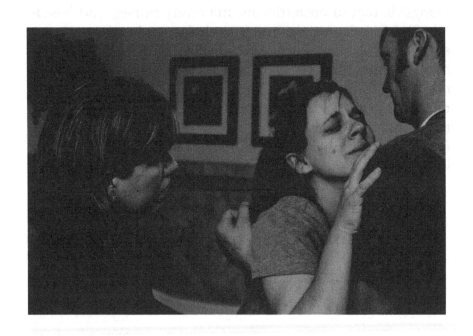

Photo 16. Doula supporting a woman and her partner during labor.
Photo by Kyndal May.

Personal Story

TURNING THE TIDE
Rebecca Flass Delgrosso

The day I toured the hospital where I planned to have my second child, I threw myself into a chair in the lobby and sobbed. I felt my dream of a positive birth experience slipping away, and I felt powerless to turn the tide. What began as a hopeful tour of the maternity ward ended as a somber march around a place that seemed to discourage natural childbirth.

It's amazing that a tool meant to sell people on the hospital and set minds at ease had the opposite effect on me. As the tour guide showed us the bed with the stirrups, mentioned that we'd be offered an epidural even if we didn't want one, and noted that we could not use birthing balls or a birthing tub, I began to fear that I wouldn't be able to achieve my goal of an unmedicated birth.

Oddly enough, it was the cafeteria hours that put me over the edge and made me the most irate. It seems a strange thing to care about—after all, what's a little food when we're dealing with the miracle of bringing human life into the world—but when our guide said we would be unable to order a meal after 7 p.m., I panicked. I imagined a repeat of my first childbirth experience, when I labored for 12 hours flat on my back in a hospital bed with only ice chips and an IV to sustain me before giving birth in the wee hours of the morning. At that time, my husband watched incredulously as I declined to hold my new baby, instead reaching for the dining menu and devouring a sandwich and drink before finally touching my child an hour later.

I didn't want to be that person again. I didn't want to be so hungry and exhausted after childbirth that I couldn't take the time to hold my child. I didn't want Pitocin, which I'd been pushed into getting the first time around by a doctor who I suspected simply did not want to hang around the hospital all night waiting for my baby to be born. I didn't want to lie flat on my back in a hospital bed trying to push my baby out when everything I'd read suggested that's one of the least effective positions. And even though I am admittedly a wimp when it comes to pain, I didn't want an epidural. I didn't like the idea of any drugs reaching my baby.

I wanted to be mobile, and I also wanted to feel the contractions so that I knew when to push, rather than watching them on a monitor and feeling like a failure when my pushes were ineffective. I had also read that during natural childbirth, the body releases endorphins that aid in helping the mother bond with her baby, and I couldn't help feeling that if I achieved that this time, I might not spend the first year of my second daughter's life crying over what I'd lost instead of celebrating what I'd gained, as I'd done with my first child.

While it might have been easier to have the birth experience I wanted at home or at a birthing center, I was too fearful that an emergency might arise and wanted surgeons and proper equipment nearby if necessary. And so, once I picked myself up off that chair in the hospital and stopped crying, I decided I needed reinforcements.

Upon hearing about my plans for natural childbirth, my obstetrician suggested I use a doula. "You wouldn't mind?" I asked in amazement, thinking she might see a doula as an annoyance, someone who might get in the way or threaten her authority. "Oh, no," she reassured me. "They make our job easier."

I wasn't entirely comfortable with a stranger being present for one of life's most intimate moments, but I realized I would get to know the doula better than the nurses, who I'd be meeting for the first time in the hospital. I also remember feeling somewhat abandoned during my first birth, with nurses coming in and out to monitor vital signs, and the doctor coming in to catch the baby, with very little support in between. Both my husband and I felt reassured that the doula would be in the hospital room with us the entire time.

My obstetrician had a list of doulas in training who would attend births for free to earn their certification, but I decided I needed someone who had been through this many times before. I wanted to break away from an assembly-line approach to birth where you go in, get your IV and epidural, lie down and push until you either finally get the baby out, or give up and have a c-section. In short, I wanted someone who could help me buck what I viewed as a flawed system.

With only a month and a half until my due date, I asked friends for recommendations, and pored over listings on www.dona.org, a website for the largest doula organization in the world. My search eventually led me to Janet, a certified doula and former nurse who had attended hundreds of births.

Since I was so far along, we dispensed with the normal meet-and-greet and went straight to a prenatal consultation at my house. I was immediately reassured when Janet walked in the door, exuding earth-mother warmth combined with an impressive knowledge base. As we discussed her role and my goals, I was relieved to discover that she was familiar with *Hypnobabies*, a hypnosis program I was using that involved listening to CDs and practicing various relaxation techniques to have a drug-free birth. The program encourages the use of a hypno-doula, but I felt lucky to have found any doula at this late stage and was just happy that she didn't laugh at me or suggest it might not work.

Inspired by books like *Ina May's Guide to Childbirth* by midwife Ina May Gaskin, and films like Ricki Lake's *The Business of Being Born*, I had formulated an idea of what I wanted for my birth experience and was comforted that Janet seemed to think we could attempt it in a hospital setting. She provided me with some handouts to aid in writing my birth plan and we met a week later at Starbucks to go over it.

I remember feeling very empowered and encouraged as Janet and I discussed the best way for me to have an easy, unmedicated birth. It was wonderful to have an ally. I was amazed as Janet agreed that I could ask to have the lights dimmed (somehow, I thought those harsh lights were required), refuse an IV so I could walk around or labor in the shower, have only intermittent fetal monitoring as long as the baby was doing okay, push instinctively instead of having the doctor tell me to do it, and best of all, eat and drink as I wished! While that last item was a definite no-no at my hospital, I put it in a draft of my birth plan, and then asked Janet if I should remove it. She encouraged me to leave it in, and suggested that if enough women asked to do it, perhaps we could change the mindset present at most hospitals. She gave me a recipe for an electrolyte drink and a handout that debunked many of the arguments typically made against eating during labor; she suggested I show it to anyone who gave me a hard time.

Janet also provided me with some statistics regarding the effects of doula support during birth, including shorter labor, decreased need for medication, a dramatic decrease in the percentage of cesareans, and forceps or vacuum-assisted births, as well as an increase in parent satisfaction and self-esteem.

At my next doctor's appointment, I was excited to meet with the midwife, Evelyn, who had known Janet for well over 30 years, and I was hopeful she would be supportive of my choices. I nervously handed over my birth plan and held my breath as she looked it over before declaring that she didn't think any of my requests would be a problem. Whew! I was thrilled to feel that I actually had a say in what would be done to my body and my child. I was still extremely nervous about whether or not I could actually pull off a drug-free birth, but I began to view the experience as the natural event it should be rather than as a medical condition that needed to be fixed with numerous interventions that could potentially lead to a c-section.

As my due date approached, I packed my hospital bag and occupied myself with tasks like preparing a basket of snacks for the nurses, something Janet recommended. I had experienced quite a bit of cramping during my pregnancy and was sure I would go into labor ahead of my due date. Janet assured me that she would be on call two weeks prior to my due date and two weeks after, although we made sure when we hired her that she would be able to provide a back-up doula in case of emergency.

My in-laws came into town, and still we waited. Janet urged me to be patient, stating that the baby should be allowed to arrive when she was ready. My due date came and went, and when my husband, Pete, innocently noted how many days I was overdue while glancing at the wall calendar at my obstetrician's office, I again burst into tears. Four days overdue, I decided to have my membranes stripped and crossed my fingers that this would not mean bringing on a labor my body would be unable to complete on its own.

That night, I bled slightly and felt crampy like Evelyn said I might. The following morning, I noticed the cramping was getting stronger and coming in waves. Using a contraction tracking application on my iPhone, Pete and I began to time them and realized they were about seven minutes apart. My in-laws took my four-year-old daughter out for the day, my husband decided not to go to work, and we called Janet to let her know this could be the day our baby would be born. She agreed that it might be early labor, and suggested we go for a walk and call her back when the contractions grew stronger.

It was a very hot July day in Florida as Pete and I struggled to walk through our neighborhood. We did this several times that morning, and as the contractions came four to seven minutes apart and became more painful, we called Janet back at lunchtime to say we thought we were ready for her to meet us at the house. She advised me to eat something light for lunch and stay hydrated while she made the 45-minute drive to our house, so I sat at the kitchen table to have some miso soup, a plum, and water.

When Janet arrived, she took one look at me and said she believed I was not yet in active labor since I was still able to walk and talk through my contractions. If we had not had a doula, Pete and I would likely have driven to the hospital at this point, even though I knew that the longer I was in the hospital, the more interventions I was likely to have.

As the heat outside was now unbearable, I began walking around the house, encouraged by Janet to use the stairs as much as possible. I listened to my *Hypnobabies* CD while I did this, drinking in the positive messages and hoping they would help me progress. Janet also showed me how to use the birthing ball to relieve the pain in my back, and applied pressure, which I found more helpful than the birthing ball. Since I was in capable hands, Pete went to the market to buy some sandwiches for his lunch and some last-minute additions to the cooler we planned to bring to the hospital. Soon after he left, I felt I could no longer walk around the house and decided to lie down for a bit. Unfortunately, once I got into the bed, I felt unable to get out, and simply waited for Pete to come home, at which point I told him I wanted to go to the hospital. The contractions were between one and three minutes apart, and Janet agreed it was time to go.

We called my obstetrician's office to notify them that we were on our way, and when we told the receptionist how frequently the contractions were coming, she shrieked that we needed to get to the hospital immediately. However, after speaking with the midwife, she said if we liked, we could first come to the office, which was directly across the street from the hospital. We frantically grabbed our bags and the basket of treats for the nurses and followed Janet to the doctor's office, where we were quickly whisked into an exam room as

I secretly began to fear I might actually have the baby right there. The midwife initially remarked that I seemed too calm to be in labor, but soon realized I was ready to have the baby and sent us quickly to the hospital, assuring us she'd be along soon.

The walk from the reception desk at the hospital to the labor and delivery room seemed to take an eternity, with contractions coming so frequently I had to keep stopping and waiting for them to pass. I quickly got into a gown, filled out some paperwork, and promptly threw up. Aha! Transition, we agreed.

In my birth plan, I requested a nurse who was comfortable with natural childbirth and was fortunate enough to receive someone who was willing to comply with all of my requests, even proactively doing things like dimming the lights, which I had forgotten about. I had to be in bed to wear the fetal monitor, and while she promised to remove it after she monitored the baby's heart rate for about 20 minutes, my labor progressed so quickly that I never needed to get out of that bed. Panicked by how quickly my labor progressed, the nurse called the midwife twice, with the last call coming as my water broke.

At this time, Janet focused on keeping me comfortable. For instance, when I complained that it was too hot in the room even after the air conditioning had been increased, she provided me with some cool washcloths, which felt heavenly.

My midwife arrived just as I felt the need to push. I was amazed at how silent the room was, with no one telling me when to push. It was exciting and scary, and, I realized, it was exactly what I asked for. I had never been offered the epidural, and, per my request, no one ever asked me what my pain level was. After only a few pushes, my daughter was born.

"I did it!" I shouted, feeling more euphoric and proud of what I'd achieved than of anything else in my life. My baby was immediately placed on my chest and I held her, gazing into her beautiful, alert eyes with amazement. I was so excited; I'd even forgotten that I planned to nurse immediately until Janet offered a gentle reminder that I could do so if I wished. Janet remained in our room for a while longer to make sure we were okay, then left, promising to visit us at home within the next two weeks.

Because I was feeling so good after giving birth, I only stayed in the hospital for one night. I remember thinking it was interesting that my insurance company would not reimburse me for the cost of my doula ($750), given that doula-assisted births typically result in fewer interventions and can end up costing less than those without a doula present. I hope that will change someday.

Afterwards, my husband and I reviewed my birth plan and realized that everything happened exactly as I wished. It's impossible to know how things might have been different had we not used a doula, but I know that with a doula, I had the exact birth experience I'd hoped for. The same could not be said for the birth of my first child, in which I felt powerless, pushed around by doctors, and so exhausted afterwards that I likened it to recovering from the flu.

As promised, Janet came to visit us two weeks after we left the hospital to see how we were doing and to discuss the birth. We let her know how pleased we were and how lucky we felt to have had such a wonderful experience. She helped make the birth of my second daughter the proudest, most empowering experience of my life, and laid down the foundation for a strong bond with my second child.

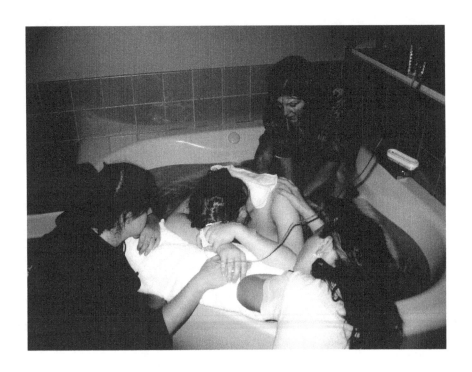

Photo 17. Doulas provide a circle of support for a woman laboring in a birthing tub.
Photo by Kyndal May.

Chapter Five

Beyond Medical and Midwifery Models: Doula Practice though a Feminist Sociological Lens[1]

The mother's womb is replaced by the womb of culture, which, comfortably or uncomfortably, cradles us all.

Robbie Davis-Floyd[2]

Doulas are one response to the encroaching technological and commoditized trends occurring in U.S. culture more generally, and in childbirth in particular. In this chapter, we examine how the history and practice of doulas helps us rethink the relative neglect of maternity support roles and practices and their role in childbirth reform in sociological and anthropological analyses of American maternity care.

Analyzing doula practice allows social scientists to move beyond a critique of medicalization per se in childbirth—to focus on the role of multiple actors as well as women's experiences with childbirth and other reproductive domains. We highlight some insights that doula practice brings to our current understanding of childbirth and reproductive domains, of calls for childbirth reform, and describe future research needed in these areas.

---

1 This chapter is based on the author's sociological research on the history and experiences of doulas in the United States. The methodology is described in the Appendix.

2 Davis-Floyd, R. E. (1992/2004). *Birth as an American rite of passage*. Berkeley, CA: University of California Press, p. 149.

Rethinking Medicalization

Doula practice not only opens up a space within existing analyses, it provides an opportunity to rethink and re-specify categorizations within underlying theories of childbirth. Most feminist and/or social science scholarship has analyzed the medicalization of childbirth, to understand the social processes by which a physician-centric, biomedical paradigm came to dominate the understanding of pregnancy and childbirth, and frame them in ways that put the likelihood of pathology and heightened risk into the foreground. Much of this analysis posits a dichotomy between the medical and midwifery models of birth, comparing their health outcomes, but also women's experience within each (Beckett & Hoffman, 2005; Davis-Floyd, 1992/2004; Declercq, Sakala, Corry, Applebaum, & Herrlich, 2013; Eakins, 1986; Fox & Worts, 1999; Goer & Romano, 2012; Jordan, 1983/1993; Kitzinger, 1989; Lazarus, 1994; Martin, 1992; Monto, 1997; Murphy-Lawless, 1999; O'Brien, 1981; Oakley, 1979, 1984; Romalis, 1981; Roth & Henley, 2012; Tew, 1998; van Teijlingen, 2005). As a result of this focus on medicalization, some researchers have pointed out that other equally important concepts and perspectives around childbirth have been unexamined. These include the changing value attributed to "natural birth" and "nature" across cultures and history, as well as the meaning and experiences of birthing women who do not fit the presumed normative model of "ideal" mothers in the U.S.: experiences of women who are young, unmarried, poor, non-white, or some combination thereof (Brubaker & Dillaway, 2009; Michie & Cahn, 1997). Another critique of the medicalization framework is that the medical versus midwifery dichotomy leaves no room to investigate the phenomenon of unassisted birth, a fringe practice that has been garnering adherents in the past few years (Dahlen, Jackson, & Stevens, 2011; Freeze, 2008).

An additional problem with the medicalized view of childbirth is that it bifurcates the issue of professional roles, leading to a focus on the midwife versus the obstetrician as the optimal caregiver for low-risk pregnant women. This approach leaves little room to consider the role of doulas, or for that matter childbirth educators, labor and delivery nurses, or allied roles, such as postpartum doulas, lactation consultants, and breastfeeding counselors as organizational and individual actors at childbirth—or as potential change agents within the maternity care system (Basile, 2012; Morton, 2009; Perez, 2012; Torres, 2013). These occupations comprise what we call "maternity support" roles: all provide information, emotional and/or physical support, and advocacy to women at some point during pregnancy, childbirth, and postpartum. Until recently, there has been little sustained research on these maternity support roles, their intersection, and differences. In 2012, the Maternity Support Survey was launched by me and several colleagues to examine three different but related roles— doulas, childbirth educators, and labor and delivery nurses in the United States and Canada, about their knowledge and attitudes toward current childbirth practices, technologies, and support (www.maternitysupportsurvey.com).

Why have social scientists interested in American childbirth not studied the experiences of persons in these maternity support roles? The answer lies partly in the gains made in the 1970s and 1980s by feminist health advocates who began to redefine childbirth as a non-medical event (Boston Women's Health Book Collective, 2011; Morgen, 2002; Reiger, 2001). Riding on the wave of influential observational studies of obstetric practice in hospital settings by feminist ethnographers (Jordan, 1983/1993; Scully, 1980; Shaw, 1974) who documented and critiqued the egregious practices at the time (enemas, shaving, straps, spinals, forceps, no family support), and the emerging interest and uptake of midwifery and natural childbirth by childbearing women in the 1980s and early 1990s, many social science researchers may have thought the battles were won. Family-centered care was adopted by many hospitals, attendance at childbirth classes was a normative expectation, and the cesarean rate, while increasing from 5.5%

in 1970 to 24.4% in 1987, actually dropped slightly and maintained a steady rate of 21% to 22% for about eight years before sharply increasing from 2001 onward (Main, Morton, Hopkins, Giuliani, Melsop, & Gould, 2011). Women's health advocacy, and a concerted national effort initiated by the National Institutes of Health in 1980, had led to coordinated policy and practice changes, including encouragement and achievement of vaginal births after cesarean (VBAC), which helped to bring down the overall cesarean rate in the late 1980s.

Another central issue among childbirth reform advocates was the elimination of routine episiotomy. The clinical evidence against routine episiotomy was strong, and, similar to efforts underway to encourage VBAC in the U.S., advocates who worked to reduce routine episiotomy incidence were largely successful (Graham, 1997). Episiotomy rates among vaginal deliveries decreased from 60.9% in 1979 to 24.5% in 2004 (Frankman, Wang, Bunker, & Lowder, 2009). Thus, many working for childbirth reform felt their actions were having a positive effect and viewed the doula role, with its promise of reducing cesarean delivery rates, increasing breastfeeding rates, and improving women's satisfaction with their births as a way to continue the gains made in VBAC and episiotomy rates.

Feminist Paula Treichler, writing just after this period, and well before the second rise in cesarean delivery rates, acknowledged these gains and theorized that de-medicalizing childbirth had an ironic, unforeseen development (Treichler, 1990).

Childbirth moved out of the private sphere, where women's reproductive and domestic labor have traditionally been positioned: more overtly visible in the public sphere, childbirth can be represented as a commodity, not only in the economic marketplace, but in the ideological and social marketplace as well (Treichler, 1990, p. 131).

Social science researchers followed this commodification of childbirth in the public sphere and began to examine practices within this new reproductive marketplace, such as assisted reproductive and prenatal technologies, surrogacy, or ideological alternatives to medicalized birth: midwifery, home, and unassisted birth. In the process, maternity support roles were bypassed as a topic of study, assumed to be subjects of larger forces rather than fruitful areas of independent inquiry.

In their 50-plus year history, childbirth educators have never been a stand-alone topic of academic study, even within histories of women's health or childbirth movements (Eakins, 1986; Morgen, 2002). Despite childbirth being one of the first major areas of "patient-centered care," researchers have largely ignored childbirth educators and their organizations, at least in the United States (Earp, French, & Gilkey, 2008). Sociologist Kerreen Reiger provides a comprehensive look at the social history of Australian childbirth advocacy from the 1960s to the 1990s in her book *Our Bodies, Our Babies: The Forgotten Women's Movement.* Her research, based on interviews with key activists and participant observation, analyzes the dilemmas faced by reform organizations in their efforts to change the management of childbirth (Reiger, 2001). This type of analysis needs to be done of childbirth reform organizations in the United States before early organizational founders are no longer available for oral history interviews. Archival documents from organizational meetings, membership rosters, etc. are valuable data sources for scholars to research the experiences of childbirth educators and their impact on reform efforts in U.S. maternity care.

Some argue that childbirth education curricula and empowerment messages around informed consent and shared decision-making from the late 1960s and early 1970s became co-opted by hospital educational programs (Declercq, 1983). Other researchers view childbirth educators as undifferentiated components of a larger childbirth reform movement that valorized motherhood above all else or, conversely, as willing accomplices of hospital co-optation (Rothman, 1982/1991), and therefore of less interest than those individuals and groups working to increase women's access to midwifery or alternative birth centers. Because the majority of social science research has explored the minority of women choosing homebirth, midwifery-attended birth, or the encroaching normalization of new technologies or reproductive practices, this has left the relationships between childbirth practices, actors, and outcomes within hospital birth still largely unexamined (Morton, 2009). However, if researchers focus attention on "the intermediate social context and social relations within which women give birth," as sociologists Bonnie Fox and Diana Worts have recommended, social scientists can expand their lens to include those roles previously neglected (Fox & Worts, 1999, p. 343). The results of such a focus, especially an organizational analysis, will likely yield important insights for birth activists around organizational dynamics and strategic political action (Craven, 2010).

Labor and Delivery Nurses

Labor and delivery nurses have rarely been a focus of social science research in terms of their understanding and views of birth or their experience working in hospital settings with a variety of birthing women (Beck & Gable, 2012; Edmonds & Jones, 2012; Regan & Liaschenko, 2007). Recent work by nursing scholars has begun to fill this gap in research. Regan and Liaschenko examined how 51 nurses cognitively frame childbirth and cesarean section (CS) rates by asking them to narrate what they saw in a photo depicting a childbirth scene. The narrative analysis "demonstrated three distinct ways in which participants cognitively framed childbirth and possible ways in which acting in accordance with these belief systems might influence the use of CS" (Regan & Liaschenko, 2007). Yet how these cognitive frames apply to nursing practice needs further investigation, as well as what happens when cognitive frames clash among the participants in hospital birth—the obstetric physician, the family, the childbearing woman, her partner, and any others.

Nurse-researchers Joyce Edmonds and Emily Jones conducted a semi-structured interview study with 13 nurses who were employed at a hospital with about 2000 births a year and an overall cesarean rate of 36% (Edmonds & Jones, 2012). These nurses work within a "nurse-managed labor model," which is characterized by a relatively autonomous nursing role with intermittent communication with an off-site obstetrician. Most nurses in the U.S. practice within this type of model. Nationally, less than 10% of hospitals that accept births are teaching hospitals that have access to physician consultation 24 hours a day, 7 days a week. Few studies have looked at nurses' role on the mode of delivery. This is more striking when one considers the many specific nursing clinical practice responsibilities that may affect cesarean rates.

Nurses are largely responsible for assessing women during triage for admission and monitoring/assessing the health of mother/baby after hospital admission. Nurses administer oxytocin, assess and assist with labor pain, and are primary managers of second-stage labor. These practices occur within the administrative context of each hospital's policies on admission in early labor, rates of interventions such as inductions (especially those for no medical indication), cesarean (especially those among the low risk population), and availability and rates of Vaginal Birth after Cesarean (VBAC).

The conclusion reached by the authors was that "experienced nurses practicing in a nurse-managed labor model have the potential to change patient outcomes" (Edmonds, 2012, p. 8). Despite the known limitations of this study—a small sample of highly experienced nurses working at a single institution—the practice implications and the potential to develop quality improvement strategies for reducing cesarean deliveries that are specific to nurses deserves additional exploration by social scientists, as well as by nurse-researchers.

Cheryl Tatano Beck, a well-known scholar in the area of birth trauma among childbearing women, has turned her attention to secondary trauma experienced by obstetric nurses; she is the first researcher ever to do so. In a 2012 study of 464 labor and delivery nurses, Beck and her colleague Robert Gable found that 35% of the respondents reported moderate-to-severe levels of secondary stress (Beck & Gable, 2012). The data for their mixed methods study included a Secondary Trauma Stress Scale, as well as qualitative descriptions from the respondents about their experiences attending traumatic births. The descriptions from the nurses in the study parallel those by doulas in my research discussed in Chapter Four. As Beck and Gable note:

Nurses frequently used phrases, such as "the physician violated her," "a perfect delivery turned violent," "unnecessary roughness with her perineum," "felt like an accomplice to a crime" (Beck, 2012, p. 8).

These recent explorations into various facets of labor and delivery nurse experience and practice are critically important; however, more research needs to be done. The Maternity Support Survey will examine how nurses compare with doulas and childbirth educators in their attitudes toward typical childbirth practices, as well as views about each other (www.maternitysupportsurvey.com). The findings from this survey will likely yield topics requiring further research, using methods like ethnographic observation and interviews (Morton, 2009). Next, we show how examining the doula role itself yields additional areas of inquiry.

Gender and the Transition to Motherhood

The doula model of care places the childbearing woman at the center, as an agent of her birth experience and also as the subject of the doula's role. Homebirth midwives also view birthing women as autonomous agents, but doulas move this model, albeit with less power over clinical care management, to the hospital. In Chapter Four, we showed how doulas utilize many strategies to highlight and prioritize birthing women's agency, even in the constrained environment of the hospital. This explicit centering of women contrasts, sometimes sharply, with how institutionalized (industrial) birth can marginalize or at times malign women's bodies and emotions (Kitzinger, 2006; Plante, 2009; Reiger & Morton, 2012). The doula model privileges the gendered and embodied practices of pregnancy (gestation), birth (parturition), and breastfeeding (lactation), by acknowledging their value and recognizing the need for supportive care as women engage in these types of reproductive labor.

These dimensions of centering women's experience in birth unsettle some feminist presuppositions or political views. One feminist critique is that the doula's claim of a unique and special female connection between the doula and her client during childbirth valorizes and universalizes gender difference, and seems to highlight women's identity as mother above all else. However, these critiques dismiss or fail to recognize historical anthropological data showing that nearly all cultures assign this supportive role to women (Trevathan, 1987).

Another often-articulated feminist critique is that a focus on birth as a transitional rite of passage to motherhood essentializes the mothering role based on biological experience, ignoring other paths to motherhood, such as adoption and/or surrogacy. Finally, informed by a reproductive justice framework, some critique doulas and their organizations for not consciously supporting all persons engaging in reproductive labor by not examining race, class, and sexual orientation issues within their training curricula and service models (Perez, 2012).

Many doulas uncritically accept that continuous labor support and "being kind to the woman" has been scientifically proven to positively impact mother-infant bonding. This notion, and the subsequent popularization of the bonding research is implicated in a wide range of feminist critiques that are suspicious of any sense that birth and motherhood are defined as the central experience for women, or that a biologically defined magic hour after childbirth is the only path for a woman's emotional connection to her newborn. The alliance of doula care with the bonding research of Drs. Klaus and Kennell raises the issue of whether doulas unconditionally support all mothers in their own circumstances and choices, or whether doulas monitor and promote an unquestioned, normative understanding of how and under what circumstances women are expected to emotionally bond with their newborns (Arney, 1980; Eyer, 1992; Figes, 2001).

The doula's assertion that the birth experience is a significant factor in how women transform into mothers—and how the couple becomes parents—highlights a looming gap in academic research on the transition to parenthood. Most studies do not look at the birth experience itself as a site for the trauma and disconnection that can occur in couples after the birth of a child (Belsky & Kelly, 1994; Gilligan, 2002; Gottman & Gottman, 2007; Walzer, 1998). Doulas witness emotional responses, verbal exchanges, and physical interactions between birthing women and their partners, friends, and family that warrant further examination of the effects of medicalized childbirth practices on the adjustment to parenthood (Figes, 2001). A national survey of new mothers in the U.S. found that 9% of the sample screened positive for meeting the diagnostic criteria of posttraumatic stress disorder, as measured by the Postpartum Traumatic Stress Disorder Symptom Scale-Self Report (PSS-SR) (Beck, Gable, Sakala, & Declercq, 2011).

Research that explores the nuances of interaction—between childbearing women and all others in the labor room—would be a source of insight into the dynamics of decision-making, empowerment, and emotional satisfaction.

Another critique from feminist sociologists who are concerned with gender equality is that recommending a strictly gendered (i.e., female) role as a support person at birth leaves little room to examine how male partners, or even male doulas, may provide this nurturing care (Basile, 2012). "Aren't doulas effectively letting men off the hook," they ask, by implicitly or explicitly arguing that nurturing is an essentially female, innate practice at which only women can excel? The majority of doulas in my study said they actively work with male partners to encourage and empower them to provide nurturing care in the public setting of birth. Yet, in the absence of a widespread cultural model that prepares men to provide emotional nurturing during childbirth, there are few frameworks to sensitize or inform men's awareness around the meaning of childbirth for their loved ones. Childbirth advice and programs directed to men more often than not reflect stereotypical models of masculinity, drawing heavily on metaphors, such as labor coach, daddy boot camp, and toolkits for birth (Leavitt, 2009; Reed, 2005). American males receive little cultural guidance or encouragement to be emotionally expressive and sensitive, and most occupations requiring emotional labor still have very few men in their ranks (e.g., childcare providers, elementary school teachers, obstetric nurses).

Another way to look at doula care and male nurturing behavior is to assert that, rather than supersede male involvement, doulas train and guide male partners by example. Doula JoAnn Ashley shares an example of how a partner's behavior changed during labor, perhaps due to her influence. She recounts how she arrived at the hospital to find her client's husband anxiously reassuring his wife. Prior to JoAnn's arrival, there had been a few incidents where the fetal heart rates were worrisome to the maternity providers. Alerted by the fetal monitor, several nurses and the midwife quickly entered the room, maneuvered the woman into different positions, and engaged in other procedures to stabilize the baby's heart rate. These episodes of non-reassuring fetal heart tones left both parents-to-be quite anxious. As JoAnn recalls:

Well, when I first arrived, Tom was at her head, patting her arm in a kind of jerky way, speaking in a tense, scared voice, saying, "It's going to be ok, it's going to be ok," over and over. I approached Carine, the mom, and said in my doula voice [Consciously lowers her voice and adds a warm, soothing tone] "Hey, how are you doing?" and just continued to talk to both of them about what had happened before I got there. I noticed after a while, he calmed down. I was stroking her head and arms with long, smooth, gentle movements, and later, I saw him doing that too. By the time they [maternity care providers] decided she needed a cesarean, she was still anxious, she needed him to talk to her. He was so romantic and described their honeymoon in Nantucket with such love and care, that both the anesthesiologist and I were nearly in tears!

Doulas tell many stories about how they support partners, as well as the birthing woman, and a quick search of doula images online results in several photos showing the doula actively supporting both members of a laboring couple. In contrast, an online search of images using the key words "nurse," "midwife," and "obstetrician" yield significantly fewer images of those roles interacting with male partners. Those images are more likely to show the nurse, midwife, or obstetrician performing a clinical task in relation to the pregnant woman. A critique that focuses only on the gender of doulas and the impact of the doula's presence on male partners ignores other, equally relevant gendered dynamics in hospital-based care. This includes gender of maternity care workers. Most obstetric nurses are female, and women represent nearly 80% of all residents in obstetrics and gynecology and approximately 50% of all active obstetrician/gynecologists (Rayburn, 2011). Indeed, it is unknown as to how or whether the increasing proportion of women working as obstetricians contributes to the trend in scheduling births and the rise in cesarean deliveries as a response to physician lifestyle concerns, especially work-life balance among female obstetricians with children of their own (Main, Morton, Hopkins, Giuliani, Melsop, & Gould, 2011). The role of gender and professional status among all actors in hospital birth settings is an important area where much more research is needed.

Race and Class: Community-Based Doula Programs

The gendered dimensions of doula care have received wide attention, however, the racial and class underpinnings of the childbirth reform movement also require attention. Doula care represents a fluid, context-specific definition of caring labor that may take particular forms depending on the relationships between doula and client and their respective identities, whether race/ethnicity, social class, native language, sexual orientation, or national origin. Community-based doula programs typically match doulas with clients based on salient identities or characteristics, such as race/ethnicity or national origin. In these programs, doulas interact with their clients in ways that affirm the shared connection of experience or identity (Gentry, Nolte, Gonzalez, Pearson, & Ivey, 2010). Whereas white doulas claim to experience a universal language of touch and kindness when working with women who come from different socioeconomic and/or racial/ethnic backgrounds, advocates of community-based programs argue that racial/ethnic concordance, for example, results in demonstrably improved outcomes (Kozhimannil, Hardeman, Attanasio, Blauer-Peterson & O'Brien, 2013).

However, there is much more to learn about the fluid, situated practices embodied in doula care in a variety of contexts, and how the doula roles of information, emotional support, and advocacy differ depending on the race or class, or even the gender of the doula and client. Doula models of care may be variously enacted within institutional settings of power, obstetric authority, and intimate relationships, and these need to be explored more deeply, especially with efforts underway to expand the community-based doula model as an answer to racial/ethnic disparities in birth outcomes (Kozhimannil, Hardeman, Attanasio, Blauer-Peterson, & O'Brien, 2013; Morton & Basile, 2013).

Beyond a Role to a Practice

A feminist analysis further suggests that doula caregiving can be more than a role–it can also be viewed as a practice. Many doulas refer to what they do as "doula-ing," transforming the noun into a verb. Doula means "to care for" in this context. The act of doula-ing exists in relation to its subject, the doula, as well as its object, the person being doula-ed. As we saw in Chapter Four, a nurse can "doula" a doula, and men can "doula" their birthing partners. In an online discussion about potty training, mothers invoked the notion of "doula-ing" their toddlers as they strained to produce a hard bowel movement. Extending the notion of doula practice to include care provision in a variety of settings renders the role (and the gender of the person occupying it) less significant than the practice of "doula-ing."

Feminist philosopher Eva Feder Kittay has gone further to extend the doula role as a practice in the realm of political justice. In her analysis of dependency relations, she argues that caring for dependents (whether due to age or infirmity) has traditionally been framed in contemporary industrialized societies as either servant/served or relations between equals. She suggests both frames are problematic because the caretaker is conceptualized as either someone in a position of economic exploitation (elder care workers or nannies) or moral supererogation (a dedicated spouse going beyond the call of duty). Kittay argues that the Family and Medical Leave Act (FMLA) of 1993, which provides for some parental leave or time to care for ill family members, fails to acknowledge the larger social contribution made by those engaged in dependency work—the contribution to the continuity, stability, and resources of society (Kittay, 1995). To remedy this, she proposes extending the doula role into a practice she calls doulia, which, in her definition, describes a system of social and reciprocal cooperation. In this way, the larger social value, as well as the varying statuses and motivations of the caregiver, are taken into account.

Emotional Support and Reproductive Justice

A longstanding concern among feminists is that caregiving, especially emotional care, is undervalued and undercompensated. In Chapter Three, we showed doula care as an example of "good women" being willing to care for others, and as a consequence, being seen as less "professional" and less financially compensated for their work (Oakley, 1993). Individually, many doulas bear the emotional, physical, and financial cost of providing a social good for altruistic reasons. Even in the most traditional form of doula care, the radical part of "serving others" arises out of doulas serving and caring for women as they become mothers. In much of U.S. culture, women are expected to do this work and in turn serve and care for their children without any particular recognition or support.

Women's psychology and social roles are organized around the presumption that they will serve others; indeed, that this serving of others will yield the only self-enhancement that is culturally accepted as appropriate for women (Oakley, 1993, p. 47).

Several doulas claim affiliation with feminist praxis and frame their work as radical—going into a medical setting with no medical credentials and placing primary emphasis on women's emotions. However, one woman contradicted the assertion this was a "safe" way to be a feminist. In her experience, it had been rather dangerous. Anna Brown sent her pregnant niece in the Midwest a copy of Pam England's book *Birthing from Within*. Her brother (her niece's father) was outraged at her actions, as the book caused his adult daughter to question things that he thought should be unquestionable—like having a physician at one's birth.

British sociologist Ann Oakley observed that the low value accorded to sociological research on reproduction was largely due to the fact that in most Western societies, women's feelings about birth are not considered important (Oakley, 1980). This critique that women's emotional experience is not a valid warrant for a specific role or focus during birth also comes from those who critique or downplay the doula's role as a change agent. There are two aspects to this critique. One is focused on the lack of doula's responsibility or influence on clinical aspects of birth or mode of delivery—in effect arguing that doulas merely "make women feel better about their births" rather than changing birth itself (Norman & Rothman, 2007). The other aspect argues that a central concern on emotional experience reflects a privileged, middle-class sensibility that is secondary to the need to address adverse health outcomes, like prematurity and low birth weight, or implement structural support for women who occupy marginalized positions due to their race/ethnicity or socioeconomic status.

Although doulas start with women's emotional experiences during birth, the expansion of doula care into other reproductive domains shows the fluidity and flexibility of the doula concept beyond its origins among white, heterosexual, middle-class women. For example, full-spectrum and "radical" doulas define their role within the reproductive-justice movement: retaining its emphasis on emotional support but consciously expanding to include support for persons of any gender, sexual orientation, race, national origin, or religion who are undergoing any reproductive experience, whether abortion, adoption, infertility, miscarriage, or birth (Basile, 2012; Perez, 2012). In the full-spectrum model, the unique, and some argue, radical, aspect of doula care is the recognition of the importance of having a caring, attentive, and culturally sensitive advocate during the delivery of reproductive healthcare (Perez, 2012). Introducing these ideas into existing doula organizations requires that members face issues of racism and other forms of oppression—conscious or not—as well as views on highly contested practices, such as abortion.

Challenging dominant cultural norms around biomedical definitions of birth can be fraught with danger—angering or alienating family members, or even other doulas—in a domain where cultural values and personal beliefs about the right, and best, way to do things are strongly held and vigorously defended. Like all flavors of feminist advocacy, but perhaps especially for nurses, doulas, and other typically "feminine" occupations, Ann Oakley sagely observes:

> … all women have to contend with one important obstacle to change: real women are not supposed to be revolutionaries … It is not good enough to say that there is something wrong out there, and we want to change it (Oakley, 1993, p. 44).

Rather than being seen as incommensurate, doula experiential knowledge and feminist analysis can contribute to one another. Doulas need to take note, as many do, that they care more about certain things at births than do their clients. Feminist analyses of childbirth can provide doulas with multiple perspectives on how meanings surrounding childbirth, emotions, and mothering are shaped by experience, location, expectation, and other factors beyond the doula's immediate control or influence, including politics, race, class, socioeconomic status, gender, and sexual orientation (Basile, 2012).

Critical feminists leery of inscribing essentialized qualities to reproductive capacities need to acknowledge that childbirth and mothering are viewed as significant by most women, with many seeing it as the most significant experience of their lives (Hays, 1996; McMahon, 1995). This reality can be acknowledged without attributing the value of motherhood among most women to false consciousness or capitulation to the patriarchy. Furthermore, when birth is the route to motherhood, the physical acts of pregnancy, childbirth, and breastfeeding can be experienced not only as a positive transformation and source of empowerment, but also as a loss, as trauma, even as rape.

As we saw, doulas and midwives have been among the first to write about the connection between women's sexual abuse histories and their childbirth experiences (Jacobs, 1992; Simkin & Klaus, 2004; Sperlich & Seng, 2008), and a significant number of women experience trauma related to their childbirth experiences (Beck, 2004, 2009; Beck, Gable, Sakala & Declercq, 2011). In addition, feminists can share with doulas and other homebirth supporters the problematic assumptions in the construct of idealized "home" birth, when for many women, home is the site of domestic abuse and not necessarily a refuge or safe place (Craven, 2010).

Humanistic Models of Birth

From the mid-1980s to the late 1990s, anthropologist Robbie Davis-Floyd conducted groundbreaking research on the experiences of women who gave birth at home and in hospitals, and in so doing, opened a theoretical window into the space between what she called the technocratic and holistic models of birth, calling that space the humanistic paradigm (Davis-Floyd, 2001). Davis-Floyd articulates 12 tenets of the humanistic model and their implications for childbirth. It is worth noting that this approach has inspired the Brazilian Network for the Humanization of Childbirth, a nongovernmental organization which, by the end of 2006, developed a program that has nearly 500 hospitals and more than 2,000 engaged health professionals (Rattner, Abreu, Araujo, & Santos, 2009).

Doulas, as an embodiment of the humanistic element of supportive care within hospital-based childbirth, have the potential to contribute to the reform of U.S. maternity care. American doulas are at a crossroads—with the possibility of expanding their services through Medicaid programs via the Affordable Care Act amid national efforts to address racial/ethnic disparities in childbirth outcomes and reduce the cesarean delivery rate, there is a clear, acknowledged need for quality improvement in maternity care (Boschert, 2013; Goodman, Stampfel, Creanga, Callaghan, Callahan, Bonzon, Berg, & Grigorescu, 2013; Sakala, 2010; The Joint Commission, 2010).

Doulas and their organizations have an opening and an opportunity to expand their reach beyond the 5% to 6% of birthing women they currently serve. Doulas provide an ethnographic window into the world of hospital birth—a partial perspective, but a window into what has long been a black box within feminist and social science analyses of childbirth experiences in the United States. Doula practice points to the contradictions, but also the complexity, power, and wisdom available to those who would listen to doulas, the ambassadors to a country still relatively unexplored.

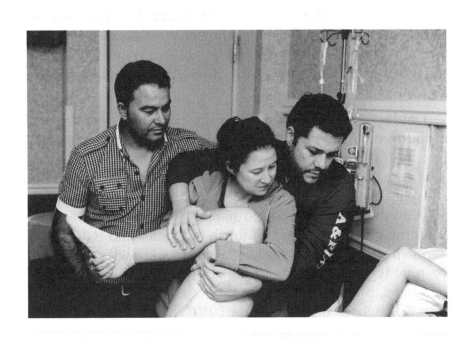

Photo 18: Full-spectrum doulas assist people in all paths to parenthood.
Photo by Vuefinder Photography | San Diego Birth Photographer

Personal Story

BIRTHING VIOLET
Ella Wilson

My mother died six months before I lay on my bed in Brooklyn and began to time my contractions.

I had never needed her more than during my labor. I wanted living proof that giving birth was possible. I didn't believe I held enough power or knowledge, enough female strength to do this alone. But she had gone, so I had hired a mother, a doula, to be my guide.

My doula, Mary-Esther Hopwood, arrived at three in the morning while I was in the shower. I had taken natural birth classes with her, determined to recreate my late mother's labor.

"I don't know what all the fuss is about," my mother said, whenever someone on television gave birth, screaming and grunting towards motherhood. I did not want to be one of those women my mother scoffed at. With her gone, her words were all I had, and so I opted for a natural birth.

I imagined I would give birth exactly as my mother had: silently, gracefully, powerfully, with wide hips and long hair stuck to my forehead. But I had neither wide hips nor long hair, and my gait tended more towards function than grace as I carved a path through my house at 3:30 in the morning with my doula at my side.

A lithe woman, Mary-Esther had the presence of a ghost, beautiful with a face that appeared to glow. She walked next to me, quiet, a sandy-haired shadow. Just as I had held my mother's hand through her illness, acting as an anchor while her body performed unimaginable feats of destruction, Mary-Esther Hopwood held my hand while my body performed unimaginable feats of creation.

Birth is, in every way, the opposite of death, but what common ground the two share is their proximity to not-life: that time before life truly begins, or after life inevitably ends. Being close to either of those states it is prudent to have a hand to hold. I had held my mother's for six weeks, and Mary-Esther held mine for what would turn out to be 27 hours. She was my anchor. She offered the conviction that I could do this. Her quiet energy flowed down her thin arms, radiating into my hands. This will be okay, your body can do this, she seemed to be saying.

Dawn came and I asked my husband to draw the curtains. I didn't want to know how long this was taking. I moved around my apartment leaning on one thing and then another. Mary-Esther, forever at my side, said little; she knew words were not what I needed. I was beyond language. Instead of speaking she joined me in that distant place that labor carves out as its own.

I wanted the birth of my daughter to be a joyous occasion. I had had enough sadness. In an attempt to insure joy, my husband and I had attended classes in natural birth. But trying to prepare for birth was like trying to learn how to be tall. All childbirth classes could offer me was a sense of preparedness. My husband and I had practiced with me rocking on all fours while he pressed tennis balls into my back. I'd sat atop yoga balls while he massaged my feet. We had squatted and counted and eaten ice chips. I had exercised my Kegels on the subway, secretly clenching my vagina while trying not to appear stressed.

My labor lasted for 27 hours, during which I barely spoke. Not because of the pain, but because I was doing something no one else could and it was demanding enormous effort: I was birthing Violet. I had imagined feeling deeply close to my husband during labor, but he seemed little more than a shadow of face, dark hair, and eyes as he stood next to me. Labor focused my mind and body in a way that little else could rival. Anything that was not essential became irrelevant. It was me, my uterus, and Mary-Esther Hopwood.

My husband and Mary-Esther urged me to eat and drink between contractions, which were coming hard and closer together. I had given up timing the pains hours ago. With the curtains closed, I had given up time altogether. I sat on the toilet with my knickers on just to rest. Mary-Esther held my bare legs, fastening me to reality. The flickering of the scented candle she'd lit made me feel sick; I kicked it over with my foot. We sat, my doula, my husband, and me, and waited.

I was on my toilet in Brooklyn having my legs held by Mary-Esther Hopwood. My mother was dead, my sister was in Scotland, my friends were at work, and my husband was a man. In that moment I loved Mary-Esther Hopwood as much as I've ever loved anyone. In the dark bathroom that smelled of smoke and wax, she held on, quietly reminding me that my grandmother had done this six times, my mother had done this, as had her mother, and in the pull of my womb I was drawn back hundreds of years to women in linen nightgowns, sweaty and medieval, the king praying for a son; women in jungles, brown and naked squatting in the leaves; women before there were diagrams or videos about how to breathe or about hypno-birthing or hot tubs. I would be one among them.

The pain intensified and the noises coming from within me changed tenor as I was guided by my husband and Mary-Esther Hopwood into the living room. A large blue yoga ball was placed in front of me, and I was lowered onto it. My knees apart, my belly hanging like a hammock of baby, my chest resting on the ball, I bobbed like a ship lost at sea. The baby was coming. I held onto the ball as if it were a life raft.

Then it was time to go to the birthing center, but I was stuck. My ankles had seized, my knees were pinned, and downwards was the only way my body wanted to go. Mary-Esther Hopwood and my husband gently pulled me up.

The short walk from my door to the car took half an hour. Every few shuffles, I gripped Mary-Esther and groaned. Her strength seemed without limit. In the car, I closed my eyes and imaged my way through the Brooklyn dark.

At the birthing center, we were met by our midwife. I sat in a rocking chair in the homey room designed to look non-medical. My blood pressure was slightly high, so I was told I'd be moved to labor and delivery. Mary-Esther stepped in front of me with the bravado of a mother, and told them to take it again in ten minutes. Then she crouched close to me and spoke in a soft voice. I do not remember what she said, but her words conjured images of softness, of submerging in cool water, of returning to calm. I listened and my blood pressure turned downwards. I registered the surprise on the nurse's face when she took the second reading.

I was helped into a wet tub. The water was warm and I lay back, glad of its suspension. I don't know how long I was water-bound, but soon I heard hard, groaning noises. As the noises changed from moans to grunts, the nurse helped me out of the tub and onto the bed. I was so close to birth that I barely felt the hand that examined me. Then I was told it was time to push. My waters broke and everything was warm.

With the next contraction, the midwife told me to push. I did, and then I stopped pushing, afraid of my own power. I looked at the midwife and at Mary-Esther, feeling panic, but they both smiled encouragingly.

I lay on the bed, my side to the mattress, one leg on Mary-Esther Hopwood's shoulder, my husband at my head, my chin on my chest, following what my body told me to do. I didn't really believe a baby could come out of me until I tried to lower my leg for a rest and felt something large and hard in the way. "It's the head," said the midwife at the look of surprise on my face. A head between my legs? Surely not, but I pushed on. I felt something pop out of me and then in one slippery moment out my daughter flew, onto my chest, and like that, I was a mother!

Her warmth at that moment of birth was as real to me as the coldness of my mother at the moment of her death. And the baby looked like my mother had–bald and helpless—but she wriggled up my chest, and gray and slippery, lay against me. Life! I had birthed Violet, and both she and I—mother and daughter—were full of life.

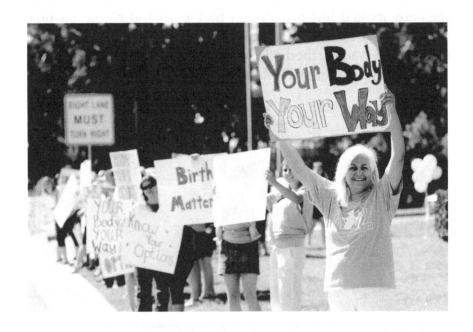

Photo 19: Doulas are increasingly involved in advocacy movements, such as this 2012 Labor Day rally organized by ImprovingBirth.org in San Diego.
Photo by Vuefinder Photography | San Diego Birth Photographer

Conclusion

The Future of Doulas

The voices that emerge in this book have been of the doulas who participated in this research, those who contributed their narratives, and our own. We have tried to open up what C. Wright Mills called the sociological imagination[1] by examining the intersections between doula care and many of the institutions, actors, and ideologies surrounding birth in the United States today: hospitals, doctors, nurses, mainstream media portrayals of birth, as well as midwives and childbirth educators, not to mention childbearing women and their loved ones. These institutions, actors, and ideologies form the structural landscape of birth in the United States. The doula, a non-medically trained person, enters the space in which these institutional and interpersonal norms and expectations play out, as a private companion to the birthing woman.

How did this happen? This book provides a first and partial answer to that question. Doulas emerged from their practical experience as women attending births, and saw firsthand the benefits to those they supported, and to themselves. They emerged because laboring women wanted them to be there, with and for them, as they birthed their babies. They emerged as a significant finding within a research study that wasn't even designed to assess the medical benefits of their presence. Yet, that study and subsequent clinical trials on the benefits of continuous labor support provided an important scientific rationale for the benefits of relationship-based, informationally open, and emotionally honest medical care during childbirth.

Still, in our society, neither women's experiences and needs nor science have justified the scarce and costly resources of time, attention, and emotional labor required to fully

---

1 And what sociologist Ann Oakley called the sociological unimagination—the discipline's lack of attention to reproductive matters except through the interconnected moral lenses of deviancy and marriage.

support and provide quality care to all birthing women. Not all women may want or need a doula, but there are many for whom having a doula makes a great difference in how they experience their birth—and their memory of that experience. While doulas may have little power to change things on an individual basis and often feel personally frustrated by this reality, it is important to know that the "private" troubles of the doula are reflective of a larger social dilemma—one in which we purport to give comprehensive, quality care to birthing women, yet fail to acknowledge that a highly technical and medical experience often leaves little room for a feeling, sentient, vulnerable woman going through a major life transition to be fully present in a humanistic way.

During an experience that will be at some points frightening, alienating, and possibly physically debilitating, doulas assuage the fear and sense of aloneness that is part of birthing. Walking into a room, the doula recognizes the sigh of relief: "Oh, thank goodness, the doula is here." Doulas normalize labor and childbirth for the woman and her loved ones who are present. They remain physically present continuously throughout labor, leaving only a couple of hours after the birth, but remain in touch until the final postpartum visit. They offer comfort, encouragement, information, and care.

What does it mean that we give birth in a culture where this service can be purchased for $400 to $800? Are we taking advantage of women who do it for little to no remuneration? Should this care, as some have argued, be provided by family or community members who will be involved in the life of the child rather than by a paid outsider? As the doula phenomenon grows in numbers and credibility, and as the real value of the doula becomes communicated—not by the doulas themselves, or by medical-outcomes research, but by satisfied clients—will we have new ideas about what form doula care should take in the future, and what position or status doulas will hold in the maternity care system?

Throughout this book, we have raised important questions for considering the doula's role in the contemporary U.S. maternity care system. We showed how historically, the creation of the doula role was a uniquely American approach designed at first to support out-of-hospital birth, but that then evolved to fill informational, physical, and emotional support gaps in the hospital setting. Doulas were the pragmatic option within a maternity care system that, overall, provides women with few options for midwifery or humanistic obstetric care in alternative birth centers. We saw that the randomized clinical trials used to support and promote the doula role largely took place in institutional contexts where women typically received little to no social support. We also saw that the dramatic effects shown in the early trials have not been realized for most practicing doulas today, leading to burnout and doula doubt.

We described the motivations and experiences of doulas, mostly women, who bring a strong desire to provide emotional, physical, and informational support to women during childbirth and a commitment to a low-intervention approach for optimal birth outcomes among low-risk, healthy women. Doulas, although avid consumers of medical research on birth, have no clinical skills or medical training (for the most part), and their simultaneous commitment to unconditionally support women's choices result in deeply felt contradictions when doulas see how choice of maternity care provider or birth setting work against the type of birth doulas feel is optimal or that their clients report they want.

Doulas work within, yet remain persistently outside, the mainstream maternity care system. There are many routes to becoming a doula, with multiple organizations offering doula-training workshops, certification, and membership-support services for those wishing to become doulas; they may work as volunteers, in private practice, or as part of a community-based program.

Much research underscores the nature and importance of social support during childbirth for maternal well-being (Mander, 2001; Oakley, 1979). However, it is not clear whether the doula, assuming an intermediary role between the woman's emotional experience of her birth, and the medical management of it, can play a significant role in fostering systemic change in U.S. maternity care. Can doulas, as non-medically trained outsiders to the hospital setting, effectively reverse rising cesarean rates and worsening maternal health outcomes? Are doulas a mere bandage on a hemorrhage, softening the potentially traumatic effects of institutional childbirth because they do not overtly challenge medical authority over normal birth and seem to accept the status quo, as some observers assert? One British scholar of supportive care by midwives offers her view that:

> The doula is nothing more than a medical answer to the needs of the medical practitioner, and the predicament which he has created in the course of the medicalization of maternity care, in general, and childbirth in particular … the doula serves no function other than to permit the continuing escalation of the medicalization of childbirth (Mander, 2001).

Since the doula's emergence into U.S. maternity care over 30 years ago, there has been a relatively stable proportion of women giving birth with doulas present (varying between 3% to 6% from 2002 to 2012), and at the same time there has been an unprecedented rise in cesarean surgery and other childbirth interventions (Declercq, Sakala, Corry, Applebaum, & Herrlich, 2013). While correlation is not causation, it is not clear how doulas, with their multiple and fragmented organizational resources, can move beyond their current marginality in mainstream maternity care culture to claim membership in the "maternity care team," much less participate in and shape the agendas of current national collaborative projects on the safety and quality of U.S. maternity care.

But perhaps it is unfair to suggest that this is or should be a goal of the diverse number and type of organizations that currently train, certify, and offer support to their doula members. Perhaps it is the grassroots nature and relative accessibility of doula training workshops, and the online visibility of the labor support role in pregnancy and childbirth social media, that is the strength and contribution of the doula, even if these contributions cannot be comprehensively measured.

Given their ideological alignment with the midwifery model of care, maybe those who become engaged in some level of doula practice are essential to raise awareness of and, consequently, increase consumer demand for midwifery care in the United States? After all, any time one of the over 50,000 persons who have taken a doula training mentions this to a friend or family member, she inevitably also has to distinguish between a doula and a midwife.[2] In this way, doulas are birth ambassadors, carrying the message and option of midwifery to an American public that is largely ignorant of the current role and the availability of midwifery or humanistic obstetric care in the United States today.

Drawing from the natural childbirth model, doulas not only contend that giving birth is a normal life event; they assert that depersonalization during labor and birth can have profound emotional, psychological, and spiritual consequences for women and their loved ones. Doulas also believe that the way society treats birthing women and the processes that babies go through as they are born, embody and create social values that are reflected in dominant understandings and representations of childbirth.

---

2 The estimate of 50,000 persons who have taken a doula training workshop comes from a communication by Penny Simkin to the authors of the 2012 Cochrane Review (Hodnett, Gates, Hofmeyr, & Sakala, 2012).

Doula practice is radical because it provides historical and clinical evidence for the personalization of birth and because it places women's emotional experience at the center of this life event. Bringing this philosophy into the hospital is risky, even in the context of patient-centered care and shared decision-making; in part because doulas assert that most birthing women are not just patients, but healthy women going through a normal, physiologic life event.

Doulas face challenges when they simultaneously assert the primacy of women's emotional needs, and the long-term social consequences for women and families when those needs are not met, within the rational economic calculus of policy makers, hospital administrators, and insurance companies who seek to reduce costs while improving medical outcomes. Asserting the rights and needs of birthing women is a strongly political action, but whether the individual acts of doula care will translate into a transformed maternity care system remains to be seen. Will doulas be ambassadors of a woman-centered, humanistic model of birth, for all birthing women in the United States?

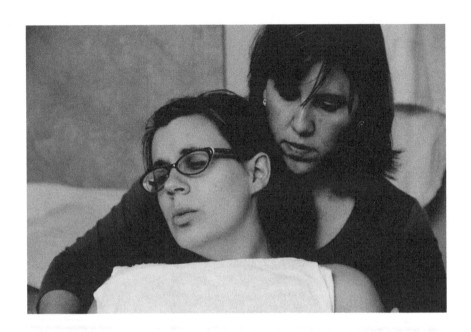

Photo 20. Doula care includes close physical and emotional connection with women in labor.
Photo by Kyndal May.

Personal Story

FROM CHANCE TO CHANGE: BIRTH AS SACRED PASSAGE
Julie E. Bloemeke

My decision to birth with a doula began from a place of chance.

In the early days of my first pregnancy, I watched *A Baby Story* on television with distanced curiosity and puzzlement. Was I like these mothers, starry-eyed over Pooh-themed nurseries, cooing over their bellies? They seemed utterly removed from me, and yet I could not help watching them.

One day, however, the edited bliss of *A Baby Story* became raw. The mom-to-be—who previously seemed so take-charge and calm about her impending birth—was now screaming behind a closed door. Her husband was pressed to the wall, helpless with shock, as nurses and doctors scurried around, apparently unfazed. I shouted at the TV: "Help her! Isn't someone going to help her?" And for one of the first times since conceiving, fear gripped me as I realized how sanitized my views of birth were. Here I was, pregnant, having never witnessed the birth of a human being. My dread continued to deepen along with a sense of fierce loneliness.

I had to keep watching. I had to know what happened.

Enter the doula. The birthing woman, on seeing the doula, clung to her with abandon, her entire energy and demeanor changed. The relief that washed over her was powerfully compelling. The doula did not speak, but placed the mother's hands behind her own neck and began swaying with her, her body slowly matching the rhythm of the laboring mom. The husband began to peel himself from the wall, while medical personnel continued their work glancing at each other with bemused interest at the transformed scene.

I was overcome. Who was this woman? How was she doing this? Then another contraction hit. The mother stiffened, pulling away from the doula, raising her soft moans to breathy, high-pitched, panicky noises. The doula calmly took the mother's face in her hands, whispered something as reminder, and brought her back to a place of low, powerful chants. She looked her in the eyes, providing affirmation, and even though I was viewing this scene through a TV screen, the intensity of what I was observing was almost too stunning to watch.

After another few moments of position-changing, back massage, hip circles on the birth ball, the pushing began. The baby arrived quickly, much to the surprise of the parents and the obstetric clinicians. But not to the doula who stood beaming at the bedside, the sheer adoration in her face almost palpable. Even though I had read copious essays, books, and writer's takes on motherhood, it was at this moment that I knew I would have a doula at my birth.

Teresa was not the first doula I interviewed, but given that my first conversation with her lasted well over an hour, I knew she would be part of my child's birth story. The first time I met her confirmed it. When she embraced me, I could feel such warmth and energy radiating from her. My husband and I began attending her birthing classes, based on Pam England's *Birthing from Within*. I was taken by how she used art, the stories of Inanna, and her rich experiences of mothering and birthing to educate us. I began to see this transition of life not only as physical act, but as spiritual connection, a place of communion with one's body, a raw, honest journey rooted in animal instinct and awareness. I found her candor about cervixes, circumcisions, episiotomies, cesarean surgeries, breastfeeding, and parenting refreshing, helpful, and thought-provoking. Of course, I did not know at the time how she would change and save me on levels I could not have anticipated.

After laboring fairly confidently on my own, and with my husband (our plan for the first stage) for almost eight hours, the panic began to set in. Anxiety was running high from all sides. This baby would be the first grandchild for both families, and on my side, the first great-grandchild, and great-great-grandchild, born almost exactly 100 years after my great grandmother. Couple that with the fact that I was at 42 weeks and had passed over the following significant dates: my own birthday (which I share with my father-in-law), Mother's Day, and both the ultrasound and midwife's estimated delivery date. Of course, had I trusted my own body, I would not have worried. I went into labor on the day I had calculated based on the formula in *Taking Charge of Your Fertility*.

But in the midst of labor, I no longer believed in this breathing, moaning, chanting, bathing, walking, hip-circles-on-the-ball bullshit. I was impatient, irritated. I needed this baby now! I was doing everything "right" and why, oh why, did it seem I was not progressing? In retrospect, I was transitioning into the next stage of labor, but was unable to recognize that at the time. I told my husband to call Teresa. Angry and frustrated, I uttered her name through clenched teeth, breathing fast and furious. I held onto a wall partition, terrified, feeling the fog of aloneness descending, growing darker. Her voice came back through the phone, firm, and loving. She breathed with me, brought me back from that luring lake of self-doubt, talked me through contraction after contraction. I felt steadied, brave enough to get to the car, and meet her at the hospital.

Once we pulled up to the entrance, I closed my eyes, and refused to open them. I was determined to stay in my head, in my body, in my place of comfort. I shut out any noise or distraction that would keep me from the rhythm of this labor.

And then, Teresa.

Already in the room, she had made it a sanctuary. She had lowered the lights and was waiting for me. She immediately came to me with her healing, reassuring hands. She swayed with me, stroked my hair, reminded me to talk to this baby that I would be bringing into the world. When the contraction passed, I noticed that she had prepared the birth ball, and she told my husband it was OK to take a walk. (His nerves had been in high-fire mode since 6 p.m., and it was now 3:30 a.m.)

She began to bring me further into a space of quiet, of comfort, but also into the work of birth. She rocked me maternally, whispered to me, rubbed my legs when I asked, held off when I did not want to be touched. She kept the blinking, buzzing world at bay so that I could enter into the sacred space of Inanna, a place of challenge, of arrival, of facing raw, animal pain, and walking through based on belief and knowing. She reminded me of my voice, to say no when I needed to, and to express my needs as they arose.

It was then that I felt I could surrender to this tunnel of purpose, feeling suddenly a part of something I have felt only then and one other time, four years later, at the birth of my daughter. Visions began to appear, of women everywhere birthing at this very moment. I saw them in huts, and in the desert, in wet rainforests. I saw women in caves, in beds, in pools of water. The more they appeared to me, the more I realized they were calling me to become a part of them, and that they were also a part of me. I realized they were women not only from all places, but all times. They were welcoming me from their place of mother—a place of survival, power, ritual, and tradition. One woman bearing her children, who in turn bore her children, who then bore her own children. The clarity of that moment brought me profound joy. This baby would come. There was no turning back. I was in the midst of birth, the passing on of us before we could continue. And then, in all of this, I began to see something else.

I now know that without the safety of Teresa, I may have not been open to this next set of events. But because she was there, loving me, reassuring me, pushing me, I felt as if I was released into something more extraordinary than I could have imagined. Suddenly my first love appeared. My place of unmitigated joy and knowing, my purpose, my call from God and the universe showed up: words. Lines of poems came rushing in, like fireflies or jewels. I could see them as they caught the sun and flashed away, almost before I could read them. Beats and breaths, cadences and images appeared from poets who have informed me, carved me, softened me, challenged me. There were words from Dickey and Dickinson, Bradstreet, Bishop, and Bogan, Moore and Neruda, Doty, Shakespeare, Mew, and Hayden. There were too many to name or even truly distinguish.

I began to weep with the intense joy, maintaining this moment of utter beauty, knowing with each contraction I was ever closer to more of the work of it, to the pushing and blood of it, to the swell and release, to the shit and scar of it. Instead of fear and stubborn independence, there was the love and wisdom of Teresa, turning me so that I could see.

In all, this place of light and poetry lasted perhaps ten minutes, but it is one of the gifts given to me in the birth of my son. It was a gift I know I would have missed had I grit my teeth and insisted I could bear through it. A gift that would have been squandered had I been left to the mercy of hospital personnel, or the random tide of decision-making from someone else, because I so needed to be in my body and not concerned with paperwork or protocol.

I could list the other miracles of my son's birth because of Teresa: she negotiated five hours of pushing for me, suggested the alternative treatment of subcutaneous water injections as a way to derail my back labor, supported my midwife, kept a random and petulant obstetrician at bay, and ultimately helped me to avoid a cesarean (a grave decision for me given my high sensitivity to drugs and years of chronic pelvic issues). And after the birth, she was determined that I be permitted to hold and breastfeed my son even though the nurses were insistent that he had to be bathed and weighed at that very moment. After 25 hours of labor, these were not things I would have had the presence of mind to fight over for myself. But Teresa saw these needs, remembered my wishes, and honored them, allowing my intentions to be the root of my birth experience.

She welcomed me into a sacred den, place of a new soul arriving on the planet, place of me arriving as mother. With Teresa as advocate, I was able to be blessed into the spiritual transition of birth, the sacredness of it, I was able to glimpse into the vastness and come back changed. My gratitude is boundless.

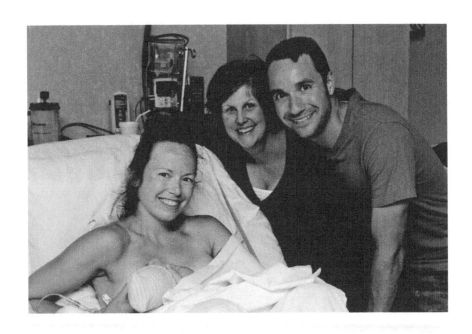

Photo 21: The happy ending: a satisfied new mother and baby with her partner and doula.
Photo by Kyndal May.

Afterword
by Mark Sloan, MD

Carved high on a limestone wall in the ancient Egyptian Temple of Hathor, a woman is captured in the act of giving birth. She squats, leaning forward, her hands gripping her thighs. Her trance-like gaze is locked in the middle distance, oblivious to a viewer's curiosity. She labors in every sense of the word, yet she is strong, calm, and even joyful: the hint of a Mona Lisa-like smile plays across her lips.

Significantly, the woman is not alone. On her left, Taweret, the goddess of childbirth and fertility, reaches a hand toward the woman's brow—a blessing, perhaps? To her right, supporting the woman's arm, is Hathor herself: the goddess of music, dance, motherhood, and joy. The three figures perfectly capture the essence of childbirth—the toil and intensity, the pain and elation, the companionship so essential to a healthy birth.

Long before the anonymous carver took chisel to stone, human childbirth had ceased to be a solo event. As the fetus and the female pelvis evolved in tandem, unassisted birth, as still practiced by virtually every other primate species, became perilous for mother and child. At some distant point in prehistory, our ancestors entered the era of "obligate midwifery," as the anthropologist Wenda Trevathan has described it; an era we have never left. Our success as a species owes a fundamental debt to skilled birth helpers.

Along with the need for an experienced midwife came the need for reassurance and emotional support during labor. For most of recorded history that support was provided by family and friends, almost always female. A circle of women cared for a laboring woman, and she in her turn provided support for others during that most female of life's passages.

And that's the way it was, baby after baby, century after century, until about a 100 years ago. Then, for reasons Christine Morton and Elayne Clift document so well in this marvelous book, the social network of women very quickly frayed, and in many parts of the world collapsed entirely. Hospital birth, with women often heavily sedated and laboring alone, became the norm in much of the United States. Centuries of cultural wisdom were nearly lost in the relative eye-blink of a few generations.

Fortunately for pregnant women, a small group of dedicated people—Marshall Klaus, John Kennell, and Penny Simkin, to name just three—persevered in the face of medical skepticism. They proved beyond doubt what human experience had long ago taught us—that the continuous presence of a birth-experienced labor companion improves every measurable birth outcome.

Their research was fortunate for babies too, in ways that Klaus and colleagues could not have foreseen 40-odd years ago. We are only beginning to understand the important role that normal labor, and the passage through the birth canal, plays in shaping the newborn's immune system and influencing future health—perhaps throughout the entire life cycle.

"Nature does nothing without reason." Sir Isaac Newton was referring to a thorny physics problem when he penned that aphorism in the 17th century, but he might well have been writing about pregnancy and childbirth. A woman protects her fetus with a constant stream of antibodies, antioxidants, and hormones throughout pregnancy, and continues that protection after birth with the immunity-boosting properties of her breastmilk.

Nature also sends a final surge of chemical and hormonal protection across the placenta from mother to child during labor; it is difficult to imagine this happening "without reason." It's difficult to imagine, too, that this surge does not have a lasting effect on a child, perhaps providing a final "fine-tuning" of the newborn's immune system in preparation for life outside the womb. We already know that babies born vaginally are less likely to develop asthma later in life than those born by cesarean section. What other hidden benefits will we discover in the coming years?

The challenge we face in the early 21st century, then, is to re-normalize the slow, patient, woman-centered approach to childbirth that served humankind well for so many generations. We have a very long way to go. With smaller families living farther apart than ever before, and the explosion of inductions and cesarean births in recent decades, we now find ourselves in a paradoxically happy and sad situation. Though modern medical technology has made childbirth infinitely safer than it was in the time of the Pharaohs, its over-application often leaves pregnant women with few, if any, female friends or relatives who have experienced a normal vaginal birth.

This is why the role of the doula—the descendent of those millions of women who gathered at bedsides around the world—is so vitally important. Some day in the future we may again reach a point where women can rely on the traditional circle of birth-experienced mothers, grandmothers, aunts, sisters, cousins, and friends to ease them through childbirth, whether vaginal or operative. Until then, skilled, compassionate doulas will ably stand in for them.

We don't know what happened to the baby born to that woman on the wall in the Temple of Hathor. We do know that he or she was born vaginally, and thus, whether she lived a few days or 100 years, she received all the benefits that come with being born in the way nature intended. And that's what we strive for today, whenever possible: the kind of birth an ancient Egyptian woman would recognize, and one that would please the protective goddesses hovering close by her side.

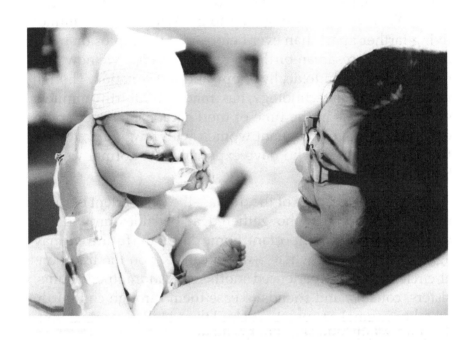

Photo 22: A new mother smiling at her baby.
Photo by VueFinder Photography | San Diego Birth Photographer

Appendix

Research Methodology
by Christine Morton

> A distinctive feature of feminist methodologies is how difficult they are to contain, how they bleed into everyday life. The borders between research and daily living are routinely and sometimes thoughtlessly crossed, only to reappear to us on the verge of publication, requiring the pretense of some traditional scholarly claims requiring us again and again to open the black box of method.
>
> Adele Clarke & Virginia Olesen[1]

The research on doula practice that is described in these chapters emerged as a result of my journey through academia, feminist perspectives on sociology, and my personal reproductive life. When my dissertation research on fetal sex identification took a back seat to the upheavals of a family move from Los Angeles to Seattle, I decided to attend a doula-training workshop for several personal and professional reasons. At the time, 1998, I had studied the sociology and anthropology of reproduction in academic settings for over seven years. This academic knowledge was filtered and diffracted through the lens of my personal experience of pregnancy, birth, and childrearing.

Initially I framed my decision to be trained as a doula as a way to put this professional and personal knowledge into useful practice. I also wanted to be strategic about restarting my dissertation research in a new locale—Seattle—that is

---

1 Clarke, A. & Olesen, V. (1998). *Revisioning women, health and healing: Feminist, cultural and technoscience perspectives.* New York: Routledge Press, p. 26.

home to an active direct-entry midwifery school and a thriving community of doulas, many of whom founded the international organization, Doulas of North America/DONA International. I figured that being trained as a doula would give me an entrée into the Seattle childbirth community that I had not been able to obtain in Los Angeles.

It helped that I was passionate about birth to begin with. The thought of being present as a new human life took its first breath was exhilarating to me. I'd only ever had the experience of bringing my own child into the world, and I was otherwise (pre) occupied at the time. While it was an unforgettable, instructive, and empowering experience, it was different somehow because it was my own. But to witness birth as an active observer—how I craved that. After years of reading about pregnancy and birth, and feeling passionately about participating in feminist scholarship on reproduction, I now felt personally, emotionally, and even physically ready to be doing something "more."

At the doula workshop I attended in Los Angeles, I became intrigued with the idea that there was a role for non-medically trained women at births and that women who wanted to provide labor support had been actively organizing for some years to gain access to and affect the outcomes of medicalized childbirth. The emotionality of the training was intense and quite a change from my academic style of learning. In doula training, emotions were considered a resource for learning and acting the role of "doula." My experiences working as a doula have been emotionally and intellectually fascinating and compelling. While practicing as a doula and reflecting on these experiences, I felt as though I had stumbled across a new discourse around childbirth that was not reflected in any feminist or social science research.

My study of doula care has been shaped by several theoretical and methodological commitments. I melded ethnographic and ethnomethodological influences from my formal graduate work in sociology with my intellectual and activist passion for feminist sociology and anthropology. In my research, I followed the ethnomethodological injunction to become a competent practitioner, actively participating within a specialized setting in order to identify the distinctive features of doula practice (Pollner & Emerson, 2001). Simultaneously, I heeded feminist sociological advice to start from women's experiences and to assume that the social organization of ongoing, concerted practices that give meaning to doula work are continually expressed in the ordinary ways doulas talk about them (Smith, 1987). In writing about this research, I have strived to follow the example of African-American author, feminist and social activist, bell hooks, whose clear expository manner belies the depth of theoretical grounding on which it rests. In other words, I wanted to write about doula practice for engaged and intelligent readers, but not bury the richness and complexity in academic jargon.

Human childbirth is never simply a physiological endeavor. The practices, meanings and social interactions surrounding reproduction are laden with cultural and political values. There is an inevitable political and ideological dimension whenever new technologies and social arrangements emerge within childbirth practices. As doulas present their role and claim the value of their care to birthing women, their accounts give meaning to and make sense of their effort. Understanding the political, cultural, and ideological dimensions of doula care requires acknowledging that every doula's account of what she does and why she does it are cultural products of particular local, and historical moments.

I do not claim to uncover "authentic" voices in doulas' accounts in and of themselves, yet I think it is important that we start with them. Tess Cosslett eloquently described her analysis of women's birth narratives:

I find myself in a characteristic post-modern dilemma: both wanting to affirm women's voices, the inscription of their hitherto marginalized subjectivities, and needing to show how these voices, those subjectivities have been culturally constructed by prevailing discourses and cultural practices (Cosslett, 1994, p. 3).

These subjectivities, including my own, are examined and analyzed with the intent of finding how discourse and practice work together in the creation and accomplishment of doula care.

For as important as discourse is in transmitting cultural ideas, equally of concern to the sociologist is how social realities are constituted in and through the practices by which members make sense of and account for their experiences. Such methods of thinking enable us to see realities as social and as arising in an ongoing organization of practices that continually and routinely reaffirm worlds in which differences and commonalities must find alliances to sustain social order. Our world is continually being brought into being as it is and as it is becoming in the daily practices of actual individuals (Smith, 1987).

Finally, I started from the premise that doulas and the women they serve are practical sociological reasoners, not "judgmental dopes"—that is, they do not enter into such a complex activity without considering its contradictions and complications (Garfinkel, 1967). As sociologists Melvin Pollner and Robert Emerson show, people are actively engaged in appraising and reasoning about the circumstances of their lives with the resulting products of such appraisal and reasoning being reapplied, in a reflexive and thoughtful way, back to the activity itself (Pollner & Emerson, 2001).

These theoretical and methodological influences were present in my attention to the ways doulas were accountable to each other for the interactional accomplishment of the ideal doula and her goal to create a positive birth memory for the laboring woman. My ethnomethodological insight alerted me to the taken-for-granted practices and features of doula work so that although, for example, I have felt what it means when a doula tells me that being at births is its own reward, I still asked, "What, then, is your reason for doing this work?" Or better yet, "Tell me how that happens for you."

Some might argue that an outsider position would have allowed me to better (read: objectively) critique doula ideology and practice, thus employing the academic fiction of putting neat dichotomous labels on complex social action. The questions that emerged from my analysis can certainly be dichotomously structured: are doulas empowering women's experience of birth or creating a new ideological demand on top of an already oppressive load? Are doulas creatively rewriting gendered norms around birth or reinscribing traditional, essentialist views of the birthing mother and the caring woman? However, my answers to these questions have attempted to move beyond the either/or and yes/no to an exploration of the individual and collective reasoning behind doula practice, not to reduce my analysis to one or the other poles of feminist oppositional discourses around childbirth.

My analysis emerged from my methodology. I occupied an outsider-within position vis-à-vis the doulas I spoke with in interviews and in everyday encounters. This position provided me with access and insight into the everyday assumptions, meanings, and practices that together constitute the social world of the doula (Collins, 1990; DeVault, 1990, 1991).

The social world of doulas consists of interactions and communications in person, in print and online; work as sense-making and interpretative practices. I have drawn on these substantially in my analysis. I employed these in an ethnomethodological sense, in keeping with the premise that:

> ... In their everyday lives, members routinely elaborate comprehensive formulations or explanations of local events, provide complex narrative accounts to themselves, other members, and outsiders regarding the ways and workings, methods and meanings of the local setting (Pollner & Emerson, 2001, p. 118).

However, I tried to be careful to recognize these as reports rather than the "real," standing apart and outside the description of the social world.

This research was based on a multi-method strategy that captured both my involvement in the doula world as a "doula" and my research objectives. The "official" data represented in this study included my attendance at three doula training workshops, as well as one doula trainer workshop, attendance at the annual Doulas of North America conference in 2000, informational interviews with eight key historical and/or organizational figures in the doula community, and interviews with 45 practicing doulas.

However, the warrant for my entry into the field and my construction of a research project necessarily occurred within the messy realities of scholarship and real life. The underlying experience of my personal practice as a doula, my membership and involvement in a local doula organization, and my participation and observations of Internet discussions about doula care all informed my formal research methods and analysis.

I encountered the intersection of ethnographic research ethics, politics, and personal experiences while defining my study. I attended my first doula training in the fall of 1998, not as an aspiring doula or as a prospective researcher on doula practice, but instead, to make contacts within the childbirth community for my study on the social uses of fetal sex identification obtained through prenatal testing technologies. After attending the training, I worked as a doula, in varying capacities, at a few births, and began reflecting and writing about my experiences. My methodological solution to the question of how I might use my personal experience as a practicing doula/sociologist to inform my research topic and analysis was to restrict the data presented here to formal interviews and observations conducted only after I decided to change my dissertation research topic to explore this world I had discovered, and which had completely captured my sociological imagination.

From January 1999 to 2002, I attended general membership and board meetings of a regional doula organization, the Pacific Association for Labor Support (PALS). I first began consulting with PALS on their website development, and then volunteered to help with a major fundraising event in October 1999. I joined the board of directors that same month. I informed the board of my intention to study doulas for my dissertation at a retreat in February 2000. They fully endorsed and were enthusiastic about the project. I raised issues that I thought deserved ethical consideration, but the group seemed largely unconcerned and were satisfied with my assurances that my data would be derived from interviews, trainings, and conferences, and not from the private board meetings or informal conversations with doulas in my capacity as board member.

My presence in the board certainly facilitated access to some of the doula population, but may also have blocked access to others.[2] My presence and participation in PALS sensitized me to many issues currently facing doulas and their organizations. In the interest of maintaining an ethical and practical division of labor, none of my informal or formal notes from my involvement in the organization are included here as "data," although again, it cannot help but be present in my analysis.

In the course of this research project, I attended baby fairs at hospitals and convention centers; I represented the local doula organization (PALS) at conferences geared toward peri-

---

2 My participation in the PALS board also may have prevented some doulas from contacting me or my contacting them. As my involvement lengthens and deepens, I have become more aware of personality issues separating doulas in this local community. These issues are complex and informed not only by personality, but diverse and differing definitions of what it means to be a "good doula."

natal social workers, breastfeeding advocates, and childbirth educators. I presented information on doulas to a class of community college nursing students.

Finally, while developing my interview guide and researching doulas, I went online to gather information. In the late 1990s and early 2000s, there was already a vibrant web presence among doulas, who were early adopters of communication and social media technologies compared to midwives and nurses. I discovered and joined a few email-based discussion lists for doulas. On one list, the participants were many and varied, representing different organizations and locations around the world but mostly situated in the United States. Another list was regionally based. I browsed websites and web-based discussions about doula care and used the themes, topics, and issues from these sources to inform and validate my ongoing analysis. I employ limited use of web-based discussions in this book.

As this research project has progressed, the Internet and use of social media has exploded. There are now a number of online sources for information about and by doulas. The Internet provides a mechanism for stories about birth, previously socially marginalized, to claim a central location in this particular topic space. Doulas collectively use the Internet in interesting and potentially powerful ways, and this deserves more research attention.

Many pregnancy and childbirth sites feature information about doulas and the doulas themselves, two of whom I interviewed as "experts" in my study: author Henci Goer was formerly the "birth guru" on ParentsPlace/iVillage.com (http://www.parentsplace.com/expert/birthguru), and now is resident expert on Lamaze International's website where she moderates the "Ask Henci" forum and appears as a regular guest blogger on *Science and Sensibility*. Robin Elise Weiss, MPH, CPH, ICCE-CPE, ICPFE, CLC, CD (DONA), BDT (DONA), LCCE, FACCE, is a childbirth and postpartum educator, certified doula, doula trainer, and lactation counselor. She founded www.childbirth.org and is the pregnancy/childbirth guide on About.com (http://pregnancy.about.com/bio/Robin-Elise-Weiss-LCCE-103.htm).

The data that comprised the basis for my analysis in this research is described below. As noted, in January 1999, I became immersed in the doula/childbirth culture in the Puget Sound area. Largely started from one local group of women, PALS has since expanded both regionally (Olympia; Island Counties; Bellingham; Tacoma) and internationally into Doulas of North America/DONA International. Many of the early founders of PALS were also founding members of DONA (currently the largest of all doula training organizations).

I chose to primarily focus on DONA-trained doulas for several reasons. First, PALS, and by extension, DONA, were among the first (and the only remaining of the early organizations) to define the doula's role. The centrality of DONA to a working definition of the doula role stems from it being the first to create viable, sustainable organizational formats for continuing to train, promote, and provide professional support for doula practice in North America (including Canada), Mexico, and elsewhere around the world. Second, due to my geographic location during this study, nearly all of the doulas interviewed were trained by DONA-approved trainers. Third, restricting the study to DONA-trained doulas provided a neat delimiter for defining a population for this exploratory research on the meaning of the doula role to the women who work as doulas. This research, then, focused specifically on the DONA definition of the doula role and doulas' responses to this role in their accounts of providing doula care.

After I completed a doula-training workshop in Los Angeles in the fall of 1998, I moved to the Seattle area and worked as a doula at six births. I joined the Pacific Association for Labor Support (PALS) in January 1999, and was certified by that organization as a labor doula the following summer. I observed one complete doula-training workshop in Seattle in February 2000, and two days of the four-day-training workshop in April. Throughout my observations of these training workshops that were attended by 44 trainees, I identified myself as a researcher, took field notes, and participated in some of the hands-on activities. When it was possible, I recorded the instructors' lectures.

My intent was to observe the content of the training workshops, so I did not focus on the particular stories of the women attending them. However, I announced my study and conducted a few interviews with doulas who attended these workshops. Attending two workshops at the same location allowed me to assess how content changed with different instructors using the same curriculum, since there is a team of instructors at that location. I also observed the second half of a training workshop for aspiring doula trainers at the end of the DONA conference in 2000. (The first part of their training session included a labor support course for aspiring doulas, which I did not attend).

I began interviewing practicing doulas in December 1999—the study includes 45 such interviews. Sheeva Hariri conducted seven of these interviews while pursuing an undergraduate degree at UCLA in Women's Studies. Sheeva had attended a doula-training workshop with the same doula trainer that I attended in Los Angeles. I was introduced to Sheeva through my anthropology mentor, Carole Browner.

Doulas were recruited for the study in both locations through announcements at regional meetings, on email lists, and through cards placed at doula-training sites. Word of mouth also resulted in a few doulas contacting us with a desire to participate. Email was the most frequent means for informing potential participants about the study and for finalizing interview details. Interviewees were not financially compensated for their participation.

In order to get at the meaning that doulas give to their practice, I utilized in-depth interviewing methodology. The research design consisted of a semi-structured interview that emerged from the questions I was asking myself (and anyone who would listen to me) about issues I encountered in my own doula training and practice. The interview guide is appended below.

Interviews ranged from 45 minutes to 4 hours, with the majority lasting one-and-a-half to two hours. Seven interviews were conducted by phone for the convenience of the interviewee. Thirteen took place either in the doula's office or a public meeting place, such as a library. Three took place at my home, and the rest took place in the doula's home. The interviewee chose the location in all cases.

Two interviews took place with a doula team in which two doulas were present and interviewed jointly. On a few occasions, children were present during the interviews, either continuously or intermittently. These included the doula's and/or my own. Interviews were transcribed, in full or in part, listened to at least twice, and were coded for key concepts.

I cannot claim that the doulas in my study are a representative sample of doulas currently practicing. For one thing, we know far too little about the current population of doulas. The doulas in my study over-represent the more experienced "career" doula. Demographic characteristics that appear relevant to doula practice are presented below.

The great majority of the doulas in my study were married (82%), while only three were divorced, separated, or widowed. Six were never married. Twelve (27%) had never given birth at the time of their interview, and all but two of these planned or wanted to have children at some point in the future. While the majority of my sample lived and trained in the Seattle area, I had interviews with nine doulas in the Los Angeles area and five with doulas from other parts of the country.

Organizational involvement was important to these doulas: only seventeen (38%) of the doulas had not served on the board of a doula organization at the time of our interview. Thirteen were doula trainers. Nineteen were childbirth educators, either certified or in training. Five were nurses or nursing students. Four were social workers. My sample included a range of new and experienced doulas, organizationally focused and independent doulas.

In summary, my sample consisted of 45 doulas who generously opened their doula lives for us to question, explore, and theorize. This allowed me to present a certain viewpoint; one I do not claim to be representative of all doulas, but one which has resonated with several who have read versions of this book and who acknowledge many of the issues that they grapple with in their everyday enactment of their doula roles.

Interview Guide

MOTIVATIONS

Tell me how you first heard about doulas and what brought you to the training course.

When did you first call yourself a doula to others / to yourself?

What is your view of birth?

Do you consider yourself a religious / spiritual person?
    Yes or No

    [If yes] How do your beliefs affect your view of birth?

TRAINING/PROFESSIONALIZATION

Tell me about your training.

    Program_____; Dates _____,

What did you learn? Was it what you expected?

What didn't you like about the training?

Have / Will you become certified through any organization?

When / Which one / Why or why not / Future plans?

PRACTICE

How long after your training did you start attending births as a doula? _____

Tell me about what you do with clients.

Prenatally   At the birth   Postpartum

Tell me about your clients

PROBES: race/ethnicity/age/language/marital status/ SES/religion

How do these things become relevant at a birth for you? For medical staff?

What is a good birth?

Give an example of a good birth.

How do you feel after a good birth?

What do you do after a good birth?

What is a challenging/difficult birth? Give example.

How do you feel after a bad birth?

What do you do after a bad birth?

Tell me about how you have worked with:

Doctors   Nurses   Midwives   Doulas   Partners   Other family members

How do you handle the emotional part of the work?

How does your partner/family view your doula work?

How many births have you attended?

_____ Total _____ as primary doula

How many births would you like to attend?

_____/month _____/year

How many births do you attend?

_____/month _____/year

If different, ask why.

How many births in Hospital?

_____ Prefer more/less/same amount?

Birth Center _____ Prefer more/less/same amount?

Home _____ Prefer more/less/same amount?

How much do you charge per birth?   (Explain sliding-scale policy, if applicable.)

How do you use the money you make as a doula?

Do you work within a practice or partnership?

Do you have a formal/informal backup arrangement with another doula?

PROBE: How reliable, how often have you used backup and why?

What sustains you as you do doula practice?

PROBES: Professional support, personal/ideological satisfaction, economic rewards, family?

What makes it difficult for you to work as much as you'd like as a doula?

PROBES: Emotional intensity, economics, family (spouse/children)?

How is doula work combined with other paid work?

PROBES: childbirth education, massage therapy, postpartum doula, "real" job?

What is a good doula?

What is a good/bad client?

GENDER DIMENSIONS

Do you think a man can be a doula?

Do you think it makes a difference if a doula has not had a child of her own?

How do you see (and how in practice is) your role different from that of the (male/female) partner?

OTHER

What do you think of the term "birth junkie"?

How do clients express their appreciation/dissatisfaction with your assistance?

Has a woman ever told you "I couldn't have done it without you"?

   What is your response?

What organizations do you belong to as a doula?

How active are you (would you like to be) in this/these organizations?

What would you like to see these organizations doing that they don't?

Tell me about how you see the history, and future of doula organizations, and the role of doulas at childbirth in this country.

DEMOGRAPHIC INFORMATION

Reproductive History

What was your age at your first pregnancy? _____

Number of pregnancies_____

Number of live births_____

Current ages of children_____

Number of miscarriages/abortions_____

What is your date of birth? _____ (dd/mm/yy)

With what racial/ethnic group do you most identify? _____

Are you a U.S. citizen?   Yes   No

What is your present marital status?
    Have you been previously married? Yes   No

Who lives in your household? _____

Please look at this chart and pick the letter that most nearly describes last year's total income for your household. Please consider all sources of income.

    a. $10,000 or less
    b. $10,000-14,999
    c. $15,000-19,999
    d. $20,000-24,999
    e. $25,000-29,999
    f. $30,000-39,999
    g. $40,000-49,999
    h. $50,000-74,999
    i. $75,000-99,999
    j. $100,000 or more

What are major sources of your household's income?

_____ (Spouse's occupation, if applicable)

What portion of your household income comes from your doula income?

What grade of school have you completed?

If college, ask for degree, subject.

Do you plan any further education?

What did/does the people who raised you do for a living and what were their educational levels?

IMPORTANT TOPICS Checklist

— Meaning of being a doula—personally / ideologically
— Integrating doula work with everyday life
— Emotional labor and its significance
— Conflicts over role (with other clinical staff / pregnant woman / partner / doulas)
— Future (personal work as doula and of the profession as a whole)

THANK YOU SO MUCH

About the Authors

Christine H. Morton, a research sociologist, completed her Ph.D. in Sociology at the University of California, Los Angeles. She attended births as a certified doula through the Pacific Association for Labor Support in Seattle, WA from 1999 to 2001. Her research and publications have focused on women's reproductive experiences and maternity care roles. She is the founder of an online listserv for social scientists studying reproduction: ReproNetwork.org, with more than 300 subscribers. Since 2008, she has been at Stanford University's California Maternal Quality Care Collaborative (www.cmqcc.org), an organization working to improve maternal quality care and reduce preventable maternal death and injury. She lives with her husband, two school-age children, and two dogs in the San Francisco Bay Area.

Elayne G. Clift, an award-winning writer, journalist, and adjunct professor in the humanities at several New England colleges, has worked internationally as a health communications and gender specialist and an educator/advocate on maternal and child health issues. A volunteer doula and former consumer representative on the Vermont State Nursing Board, books she has conceived and edited include *Women, Philanthropy and Social Change: Visions for a Just Society* (UPNE/Tufts University, 2007) and *Women's Encounters with the Mental Health Establishment: Escaping the Yellow Wallpaper* (Haworth Press, 2002). A Vermont Humanities Scholar, she has also published fiction, poetry, and memoir. She lives with her husband in Saxtons River, Vermont.

About the Contributors

Emme Dague Amble is a writer, photographer, and most importantly, a mama to four. She is passionate about her family, living life to the fullest, and helping others to tell their truth boldly. She believes that giving birth four times is both a gift and her greatest accomplishment.

Julie E. Bloemeke is the mother of two children, both welcomed into the world through doula-assisted births. Her poetry has appeared in numerous anthologies and journals, and she is a guest blogger for Best American Poetry. She currently lives in Alpharetta, Georgia. She dedicates this essay with tremendous gratitude and reverence to her doulas and spiritual mothers, Teresa Howard and Guina Bixler.

Rebecca Flass Delgrosso is a journalist turned stay-at-home mom. She has written for several business and trade publications, such as *The Los Angeles Business Journal, Adweek,* and *PR Week.* She lives in Ponte Vedra Beach, FL with her husband and two daughters.

Ellen Derby is a wife and mother of four. She has been a doula since 2002. An advocate for birthing women and breastfeeding, she is an avid needle crafter.

Kelly Martineau is a writer of memoir essays. She holds an MFA in Creative Writing from Spalding University, and lives in Seattle with her husband and daughter.

Carol Schnabel is the mother of two young men who were born at home with the support of their father, midwives, and friends. She is a volunteer doula and a professional weaver in Guilford, Vermont.

Ella Wilson, a writer and creative director of an advertising agency, received her MFA in Creative Writing from The New School in 2009. She lives with her husband and two children in Brooklyn, New York.

Liz Wilson, a lacrosse coach and program director, was inducted into the Ohio Lacrosse Hall of Fame in 2005. A permanent resident of Timonium, Maryland, she lived for a year in Costa Rica with her three children while "embracing the opportunity of living internationally in a unique, healing, and nature-centered community." Her contribution to this anthology is dedicated to her late husband, John Griffith.

Holly Powell Kennedy, CNM, Ph.D., FACNM, FAAN, is an internationally known midwifery researcher and the Varney Professor of Midwifery at Yale University. She is past-president of the American College of Nurse-Midwives (ACNM), the professional association representing Certified Nurse-Midwives and Certified Midwives in the United States. Dr. Kennedy received a diploma in nursing from Miami Valley Hospital School of Nursing in Dayton, Ohio; a bachelor's degree from Chaminade University in Honolulu, Hawai'i; a master's degree as a family nurse practitioner from the Medical College of Georgia, a certificate of midwifery from the Frontier School of Midwifery & Family Nursing in Hyden, Kentucky, and a doctorate in nursing from the University of Rhode Island. She has held academic positions at the University of Rhode Island and most recently at the University of California, San Francisco. She holds visiting faculty appointments at King's College, London, and the University of Basel, Switzerland.

Mark Sloan, MD, FAAP, is a pediatrician and a Fellow of the American Academy of Pediatrics for more than 25 years. He graduated from the University of Notre Dame in 1975 with a biology degree, and received his MD degree from the University of Illinois in Chicago in 1979. Following pediatric residency training at the University of Michigan, he joined The Permanente Medical Group in Sacramento, California, in 1982. Since 1990, he has practiced with The Permanente Medical Group in Santa Rosa, California, where he served as Chief of Pediatrics from 1997 to 2002. He is the author of *Birth Day: A Pediatrician Explores the Science, the History, and the Wonder of Childbirth* (Ballantine Books, 2009).

Kyndal May, MFA, CD(DONA), BDT(DONA), LCCE, is a storyteller and facilitator; a confidence and community builder for expectant parents, doulas, and childbirth educators. To see more of her birth photography and learn about her childbirth education curriculum platform or her birth doula workshops, visit Baby Bump Services (www.babybumpservices.com.)

Catie Stephens is a wife, mom to two kids, birth photographer and active member in the San Diego Birth Community. She has loved photography since her early teens, and with her Dad's encouragement, pursued a career in photography. Her passion is to document the most precious moments, deep relationships and raw emotion at each birth journey she witnesses. Vuefinder Photography | San Diego Birth Photographer (www.vuefinderphotography.com).

References

Abel, E. K., & Nelson, M. K. (1990). *Circles of care: Work and identity in women's lives.* Albany, NY: State University of New York Press.

Adams, A. E. (1994). *Reproducing the womb: Images of childbirth in science, feminist theory, and literature.* Ithaca, NY: Cornell University Press.

Amnesty International. (2010). *Deadly delivery: The maternal health care crisis in the USA.* London: Amnesty International Secretariat.

Annas, G. J. (1989 [1975]). *The rights of patients: The ACLU guide to patient rights.* Carbondale, IL: Southern Illinois University Press.

Arney, W. R. (1980). Maternal-infant bonding: The politics of falling in love with your child. *Feminist Studies, 6*(30), 547-570.

Arney, W. R. (1982). *Power and the profession of obstetrics.* Chicago: University of Chicago Press.

Association of Women's Health Obstetric and Neonatal Nurses (AWHONN). (2010). *Guidelines for professional registered nurse staffing for perinatal units.* Washington, D.C.: Association of Women's Health, Obstetric and Neonatal Nurses.

Ballen, L. E., & Fulcher, A. J. (2006). Nurses and doulas: Complementary roles to provide optimal maternity care. *Journal of Obstetric, Gynecologic, and Neonatal Nursing, 35,* 304-311.

Basile, M. (2012). *Reproductive justice and childbirth reform: Doulas as agents of social change.* Ph.D thesis, University of Iowa, Iowa City.

Beck, C. T. (2004). Birth trauma: In the eye of the beholder. *Nursing research, 53*(1), 28-35.

Beck, C. T. (2009). Birth trauma and its sequelae. [Review]. *Journal of Trauma & Dissociation, 10*(2), 189-203. doi: 10.1080/15299730802624528

Beck, C. T., & Gable, R. K. (2012). A mixed methods study of secondary traumatic stress in labor and delivery nurses. *Journal of Obstetric, Gynecologic, and Neonatal Nursing, 41*(6), 747-760. doi: 10.1111/j.1552-6909.2012.01386.x

Beck, C. T., Gable, R. K., Sakala, C., & Declercq, E. (2011). Posttraumatic stress disorder in new mothers: Results from a two-stage U.S. national survey. *Birth, 38*(3), 216-227.

Beckett, K., & Hoffman, B. (2005). Challenging medicine: Law, resistance, and the cultural politics of childbirth. *Law and Society Review, 39*(1), 125-169.

Belsky, J., & Kelly, J. (1994). *The transition to parenthood: How a first child changes a marriage.* New York: Delacorte Press.

Berry, L. M. (1988). Realistic expectations of the labor coach. *Journal of Obstetric, Gynecologic, and Neonatal Nursing, Sept/Oct*, 354-355.

Bertsch, T. D., Nagashima-Whalen, L., Dykeman, S., Kennell, J. H., & McGrath, S. K. (1990). Labor support by first-time fathers: Direct observations with a comparison to experienced doulas. *Journal of Psychosomatics in Obstetrics and Gynaecology, 11*, 251-260.

Birkland, D., & Green, S. J. (2001). Survey: 23% of women say they've been raped, *Seattle Times*.

Block, J. (2007). *Pushed: The painful truth about childbirth and modern maternity care*. Cambridge, MA: Da Capo Press.

Blue, D. (1994). The re-emergence of social support for child-bearing women. *Journal of the International Childbirth Education Association, 9*(2), 29-30.

Bobel, C. (2002). *The paradox of natural mothering*. Philadelphia: Temple University Press.

Bogdan, J. C. (1978). Care or cure? Childbirth practices in nineteenth century America. *Feminist Studies, 4*, 92-99.

Boschert, S. (2013, 7/7/13). Maternity safety blueprint outlined, *Ob-Gyn News*. Retrieved from http://www.obgynnews.com/news/top-news/single-article/maternal-safety-blueprint-outlined/80ca51a7604a-9320b757557e65c0fe88.html.

Boston Women's Health Book Collective. (2011). *Our bodies, ourselves*. New York: Touchstone.

Bowser, D., & Hill, K. (2010). Exploring evidence for disrespect and abuse in facility-based childbirth: Report of a landscape analysis. In United States Agency for International Development (Ed.), *Translating Research Into Action*. Cambridge, MA: Harvard School of Public Health, University Research Co., LLC.

Braddock, C., Edwards, K., Hasenberg, N., Laidley, T., & Levinson, W. (1999). Informed decision making in outpatient practice: Time to get back to basics. *Journal of the American Medical Association, 282*(24), 2313-2320.

Bridges, K. M. (2011). *Reproducing race: An ethnography of pregnancy as a site of racialization.* Berkeley, CA: University of California Press.

Brockenbrough, M. (2000). *Doula unto others.* [Web log post.] Retrieved from: http://womencentral.msn.com/family/pregnancy/pregnancyweek3.asp [No longer available online].

Brubaker, S. J., & Dillaway, H. E. (2009). Medicalization, natural childbirth and birthing experiences. *Sociology Compass, 3*(1), 31-48.

Budin, W. C. (2007). Care practices that support normal birth. *The Journal of Perinatal Education, 16*(3), 1-2.

Cassidy, T. (2006). *Birth: The surprising history of how we are born.* New York: Atlantic Monthly Press.

Caton, D. (1999). *What a blessing she had chloroform: The medical and social response to the pain of childbirth from 1800 to the present.* New Haven, CT: Yale University Press.

Chambliss, D., F. (1996). *Beyond caring: Hospitals, nurses and the social organization of ethics.* Chicago: University of Chicago Press.

Clarke, A., & Olesen, V. (1998). *Revisioning women, health and healing: Feminist, cultural and technoscience perspectives.* New York: Routledge Press.

Coburn, D., Rappolt, S., Bourgeault, I., & Angus, J. (1999). *Medicine, nursing and the state.* Ontario, Canada: Garamond Press.

Collins, P. H. (1990). *Black feminist thought: Knowledge, consciousness and the politics of empowerment.* Boston: Unwin Hyman.

Cosslett, T. (1994). *Women writing childbirth: Modern discourses of motherhood.* Manchester, UK: Manchester University Press.

Cowan, N. M., & Cowan, R. S. (1996). *Our parents' lives: Jewish assimilation in everyday life.* New Brunswick, NJ: Rutgers University Press.

Craven, C. (2010). *Pushing for midwives: Homebirth mothers and the reproductive rights movement.* Philadelphia, PA: Temple University Press.

Dahlen, H., Jackson, M., & Stevens, J. (2011). Homebirth, free-birth and doulas: Casualty and consequences of a broken maternity system. *Women and Birth, 24,* 47-50. doi: 10.1016/j.wombi.2010.11.002

Davies, B., & Hodnett, E. (2002). Labor support: Nurses' self-efficacy and views about factors influencing implementation. *Journal of Obstetric, Gynecologic, and Neonatal Nursing, 31*(1), 48-56.

Davis, E., & Pascali-Bonaro, D. (2010). *Orgasmic birth: Your guide to a safe, satisfying and pleasurable birth experience.* New York: Rodale Books.

Davis-Floyd, R. E. (1992/2004). *Birth as an American rite of passage.* Berkeley, CA: University of California Press.

Davis-Floyd, R. E. (2001). The technocratic, humanistic, and holistic paradigms of childbirth. *International Journal of Gynecology and Obstetrics, 75* (Supplement 1), S5-S23.

Davis-Floyd, R. E., & St John, G. (1998). *From doctor to healer: The transformative journey.* New Brunswick, NJ: Rutgers University Press.

Declercq, E. (1983). The politics of co-optation: Strategies for childbirth educators. *Birth, 10*(3), 167-172.

Declercq, E. (2012). Trends in midwife-attended births in the United States, 1989-2009. *Journal of Midwifery & Women's Health, 57*(4), 321-326. doi: 10.1111/j.1542-2011.2012.00198.x

Declercq, E., Sakala, C., Corry, M. P., Applebaum, S., & Herrlich, A. (2013). *Listening to Mothers III: Pregnancy and childbirth*. New York: Childbirth Connection.

Deitrick, L., & Draves, P. R. (2008). Attitudes towards doula support during pregnancy by clients, doulas and labor-and-delivery nurses: A case study from Tampa, Florida. *Human Organization, 67*(4), 397-406.

DeVault, M. L. (1990). Talking and listening from women's standpoint: Feminist strategies for interviewing and analysis. *Social Problems, 37*(1), 96-115.

DeVault, M. L. (1991). *Feeding the family: The social organization of caring as gendered work*. Chicago: University of Chicago Press.

Diamond, S. L. (1998). *Hard labor: Reflections of an obstetrical nurse*. New York: Forge Press.

Donegan, J. B. (1978). *Women and men midwives: Medicine, morality, and misogyny in early America*. Westport, CT: Greenwood Press.

Donnison, J. (1977). *Midwives and medical men: A history of inter-professional rivalries and women's rights*. New York: Schocken Press.

Doran, L., & Caron, L. (2010). *Bearing witness: Childbirth stories told by doulas*. Kingston, Ontario: Fox Women's Books.

Doran, L., & Caron, L. (2012). *Joyful birth: More childbirth stories told by doulas*. Kingston, Ontario: Fox Women's Books.

Eakins, P. S. (1984). The rise of the free standing birth center: Principles and practice. *Women and Health, 9*(4), 49-64.

Eakins, P. S. (1986). *The American way of birth*. Philadelphia: Temple University Press.

Earp, J. A. L., French, E. A., & Gilkey, M. B. (2008). *Patient advocacy for health care quality: Strategies for achieving patient-centered care*. Sudbury, MA: Jones and Bartlett.

Edmonds, J. K., & Jones, E. (2012). Intrapartum nurses' perceived influence on birth mode decisions and outcomes. *Journal of Obstetric, Gynecological, and Neonatal Nursing, 42,* 3-11. doi: DOI: 10.1111/j.1552-6909.2012.01422.x

Edwards, M., & Waldorf, M. (1984). *Reclaiming birth: History and heroines of American childbirth reform*. Trumansburg, NY: The Crossing Press Summer.

Eftekhary, S., Klein, M. C., & Xu, S. Y. (2010). The life of a Canadian doula: Successes, confusion, and conflict. *Journal of Obstetrics and Gynaecology Canada, 32*(7), 642-649.

England, P. (2000). What are you bringing to birth? PALS Papers: *A Quarterly Publication of the Pacific Association for Labor Support, Summer.*

Enkin, M., Keirse, M., Neilson, J., Crowther, C., Duley, L., Hodnett, E., & Hofmeyr, J. (2000). *A guide to effective care in pregnancy and childbirth* (Third Edition). New York: Oxford University Press.

Epstein, R. H. (2010). *Get me out: A history of childbirth from the garden of Eden to the sperm bank*. New York: W.W. Norton and Company.

Eyer, D. (1992). *Mother-infant bonding: A scientific fiction*. New Haven: Yale University Press.

Faldet, R., & Fitton, K. (1997). *Our stories of miscarriage: Healing with words*. Minneapolis: Fairview Press.

Figes, A. (2001). *Life after birth: What your friends won't tell you about motherhood*. New York: St. Martin's Press.

Finch, J., & Groves, D. (1983). *A labour of love: Women, work and caring*. Boston: Routledge and Kegan Paul.

Fisher, B. (1990). Alice in the human services: A feminist analysis of women in the caring professions. In E. K. Abel & M. K. Nelson (Eds.), *Circles of care: Work and identity in women's lives* (pp. 108-131). Albany, NY: State University of New York Press.

Fisher, B., & Tronto, J. (1990). Toward a feminist theory of caring. In E. K. Abel & M. K. Nelson (Eds.), Circles of care: *Work and identity in women's lives* (pp. 35-62). Albany, NY: State University of New York Press.

Fleischman, A. R. (2011). *Can we prevent non-medically indicated early deliveries?* Paper presented at the Midwest Business Group on Health Summit on Preventing Unnecessary Early Deliveries. Chicago, IL. Retrieved from http://www.hhco.org/

Fox, B., & Worts, D. (1999). Revisiting the critique of medicalized childbirth: A contribution to the sociology of birth. *Gender and Society, 13*, 326-346.

Francis, L. E., Berger, C. S., & Kim, K. (2008). Emotion and inequality in maternity care: Anguish and anger in prenatal services for the poor. In J. Robinson & D. T. Clay-Warner (Eds.), *Social structure and emotion* (pp. 343-355). New York: Elsevier.

Frankman, E. A., Wang, L., Bunker, C. H., & Lowder, J. L. (2009). Episiotomy in the United States: Has anything changed? *American Journal of Obstetrics and Gynecology, 200*(5), e571-577. doi: 10.1016/j.ajog.2008.11.022

Freeze, R. A. S. (2008). *Born free: Unassisted childbirth in North America.* Ph.D, thesis. University of Iowa, Iowa City.

Gagnon, A. J., & Waghorn, K. (1996). Supportive care by maternity nurses: A work sampling study in an intrapartum unit. *Birth, 23*(1), 1-21.

Gagnon, A. J., Waghorn, K., & Covell, C. (1997). A randomized trial of one-to-one nurse support of women in labor. *Birth, 24*(2), 71-77.

Garfinkel, H. (1967). *Studies in ethnomethodology.* Cambridge: Polity Press.

Gaskin, I. M. (1977/1990). *Spiritual midwifery.* Summertown, TN: The Book Publishing Company.

Gaskin, I. M. (2003). *Ina May's guide to childbirth.* New York: Bantam.

Gentry, Q. M., Nolte, K. M., Gonzalez, A., Pearson, M., & Ivey, S. (2010). "Going beyond the call of doula": A grounded-theory analysis of the diverse roles community-based doulas play in the lives of pregnant and parenting adolescent mothers. *The Journal of Perinatal Education, 19*(4), 24-40. doi: 10.1624/105812410X530910

Giglio, A.-M. (1999). *Labor day: Shared experiences from the delivery room.* New York: Workman Publishing Company.

Gilligan, C. (2002). *The birth of pleasure.* New York: Knopf.

Gilliland, A. L. (2011). After praise and encouragement: Emotional support strategies used by birth doulas in the USA and Canada. *Midwifery, 27*(4), 342, 525-531. doi: 10.1016/j.midw.2010.04.006

Glenn, A. W. (2013). *Birth, breath and death: Meditations on motherhood, chaplaincy and life as a doula.* Publisher: A.W. Glenn.

Goer, H. (1995). *Obstetric myths versus research realities.* New York: Bergin and Garvey.

Goer, H. (2004). Humanizing birth: A global grassroots movement. *Birth, 31*(4), 308-314.

Goer, H., & Romano, A. (2012). *Optimal care in childbirth: The case for a physiological approach.* Seattle, WA: Classic Day Publishing.

Goodman, D., Stampfel, C., Creanga, A. A., Callaghan, W. M., Callahan, T., Bonzon, E., Berg, C.J., & Grigorescu, V. (2013). Revival of a core public health function: State- and urban-based maternal death review processes. *Journal of Women's Health.* doi: 10.1089/jwh.2013.4318

Gordon, N. P., Walton, D., McAdam, E., Derman, J., Gallitero, G., & Garrett, L. (1999). Effects of providing hospital-based doulas in health maintenance organization hospitals. *Obstetrics and Gynecology, 93*(3), 422-426.

Gordon, S., Benner, P., & Noddings, N. (1996). *Caregiving: Readings in knowledge, practice, ethics, and politics.* Philadelphia: University of Pennsylvania Press.

Gottman, J., & Gottman, J. S. (2007). *And baby makes three: The six-step plan for preserving marital intimacy and rekindling romance after baby arrives.* New York: Three Rivers Press.

Graham, I. D. (1997). *Episiotomy: Challenging obstetric interventions*. Oxford: Blackwell Science Inc.

Gurevich, R. (2000). *Fabjob.com guide to become a doula*. Calgary: Fabjob.com Ltd.

Gurman, T. A., & Becker, D. (2008). Factors affecting Latina immigrants' perceptions of maternal health care: Findings from a qualitative study. *Health Care for Women International, 29*(5), 507-526.

Harrison, M. (1982). *A woman in residence*. New York: Random House.

Hays, S. (1996). *The cultural contradictions of motherhood*. New Haven, CT: Yale University Press.

Hochschild, A. R. (1983). *The managed heart: Commercialization of human feeling*. Berkeley, CA: University of California Press.

Hodnett, E. D. (1997). Commentary: Are nurses effective providers of labor support? Should they be? Can they be? *Birth, 24*(2), 78-80.

Hodnett, E. D. (1999). *Caregiver support for women during childbirth*. Oxford: Cochrane Library.

Hodnett, E. D., Gates, S., Hofmeyr, G. J., & Sakala, C. (2012). Continuous support for women during childbirth. *Cochrane Database of Systematic Reviews, 10*(Art. No.: CD003766). doi: DOI: 10.1002/14651858.CD003766.pub4

Hodnett, E. D., Lowe, N. K., Hannah, M. E., & Gagnon, A. J. (2003). Continuous labour support by a nurse did not reduce the rate of cesarean delivery. *Evidence-based Obstetrics and Gynecology, 5*(1), 8-9.

Hodnett, E. D., & Osborn, R. (1989a). Effects of continuous intrapartum professional support on childbirth outcomes. *Research in Nursing and Health, 12*(5), 289-297.

Hodnett, E. D., & Osborn, R. (1989b). A randomized trial of the effects of *monitrice* support during labor: Mother's views two to four weeks postpartum. *Birth, 16*(4), 177-184.

Hodnett, E. D., Stremler, R., Willan, A. R., Weston, J. A., Lowe, N. K., Simpson, K. R., . . . Gafni, A. (2009). Effect on birth outcomes of a formalized approach to care in hospital labor assessment units: International, randomized controlled trial. *Obstetrical and Gynecological Survey, 64*(2), 82-83.

Hrdy, S. B. (1999). *Mother nature: A history of mothers, infants and natural selection.* New York: Pantheon.

Hunter, B., & Deery, R. (Eds.). (2008). *Emotions in midwifery and reproduction.* Hampshire, England: Palgrave Macmillan.

Jacobs, J. L. (1992). Child sexual abuse victimization and later sequelae during pregnancy and childbirth. *Journal of Child Sexual Abuse, 1*(1), 103-112.

James, V., & Gabe, J. (1996). *Health and the sociology of emotions.* Oxford, UK: Blackwell Publishers.

Johnson, N. (2010, December 26). As early elective deliveries increase so do health risks for mother, child, *MercuryNews.com.* Retrieved from http://www.mercurynews.com/news/ci_16943085?nclick_check=1

Johnson, S. (1999). *A better woman: A memoir.* New York: Washington Square Press.

Jordan, B. (1983/1993). *Birth in four cultures: A cross-cultural investigation of childbirth in Yucatan, Holland, Sweden and the United States.* Prospect Heights, IL: Waveland Press.

Jordan, E. T., Van Zandt, S. E., & Wright, E. (2008). Doula care: Nursing students gain additional skills to define their professional practice. *Journal of Professional Nursing, 24*(2), 118-121. doi: 10.1016/j.profnurs.2007.06.018

Kahn, R. P. (1995). *Bearing meaning: The language of birth.* Urbana, IL: University of Illinois Press.

Kennell, J. H., Klaus, M. H., McGrath, S. K., Robertson, S. S., & Hinkley, C. (1991). Continuous emotional support during labor in a US hospital: A randomized controlled trial. *JAMA: The Journal of the American Medical Association, 265*(17), 2197-2201.

Kittay, E. F. (1995). Taking dependency seriously: The Family and Medical Leave Act considered in the light of the social organization of dependency work and gender equality. *Hypatia, 10*, 8-22.

Kitzinger, S. (1989). *Giving birth: How it really feels.* New York: The Noonday Press.

Kitzinger, S. (2006). *Birth crisis.* New York: Routledge.

Klassen, P. E. (2001). *Blessed events: Religion and home birth in America.* Princeton, NJ: Princeton University Press.

Klaus, M. H., Jerauld, H., Kreger, N., McAlpine, W., Steffa, M., & Kennell, J. H. (1972). Maternal attachment: Importance of the first postpartum days. *New England Journal of Medicine, 286*(9), 460-463.

Klaus, M. H., Kennell, J. H., & Klaus, P. H. (1993). *Mothering the mother: How a doula can help you have a shorter, easier and healthier birth.* Reading, MA: Addison Wesley Publishing Company.

Klaus, M. H., Kennell, J. H., Robertson, S. S., & Sosa, R. (1986). Effects of social support during parturition on maternal and infant morbidity. *British Medical Journal, 293*(6547), 585-587.

Klein, M. C., Kaczorowski, J., Hall, W. A., Fraser, W., Liston, R. M., Eftekhary, S., . . . Chamberlaine, A. (2009). The attitudes of Canadian maternity care practitioners towards labour and birth: many differences but important similarities. *Journal of Obstetrics and Gynaecology Canada, 31*(9), 827-840.

Kolder, V. E. B., Gallagher, J., & Parsons, M. T. (1987). Court-ordered obstetrical interventions. *New England Journal of Medicine, 316*, 1192-1196.

Korst, L. M. (2012). *Why birth plans don't work...and how they can: Your step-by-step guide to a safe and confident childbirth.* Publisher: L.M. Korst.

Korst, L. M., Eusebio-Angeja, A. C., Chamorro, T., Aydin, C. E., & Gregory, K. D. (2003). Nursing documentation time during implementation of an electronic medical record. *Journal of Nursing Administration, 33*(1), 24-30.

Koumouitzes-Douvia, J., & Carr, C. A. (2006). Women's perceptions of their doula support. *The Journal of Perinatal Education, 15*(4), 34-40. doi: 10.1624/105812406X151402

Kozhimannil, K., Hardeman, R., Attanasio, L., Blauer-Peterson, C., & O'Brien, M. (2013). Doula care, birth outcomes, and costs among Medicaid beneficiaries. *American Journal of Public Health, 103*(4), e113-121. doi: doi:10.2105/AJPH.2012.301201

Lake, R., Epstein, A., & Mortiz, J. (2010). *Your best birth: Know all your options, discover the natural choices, and take back the birth experience.* New York: Grand Central Life & Style.

Lantz, P. M., Low, L. K., Varkey, S., & Watson, R. L. (2005). Doulas as childbirth paraprofessionals: Results from a national survey. *Women's Health Issues, 15*(3), 109-116. doi: 10.1016/j.whi.2005.01.002

Lazarus, E. S. (1994). What do women want?: Issues of choice, control and class in pregnancy and childbirth. *Medical Anthropology Quarterly, 8*(1), 25-46.

Leavitt, J. W. (1986). *Brought to bed: Childbearing in America, 1750-1950.* Oxford, UK: Oxford University Press.

Leavitt, J. W. (2009). *Make room for Daddy: The journey from waiting room to birthing room.* Chapel Hill, NC: The University of North Carolina Press.

Lemay, G. (2008, November 18). *Collecting money for our work.* [Web log post]. Retrieved from http://www.glorialemay.com/blog/?p=54; accessed 10/28/12

Lewis, J. (1986). *In the family way: Childbearing in the British aristocracy, 1760-1860.* New Brunswick, NJ: Rutgers University Press.

Litt, J. S. (2000). *Medicalized motherhood: Perspectives from the lives of African-American and Jewish women.* New Brunswick, NJ: Rutgers University Press.

Lu, M. C., Prentice, J., Yu, S. M., Inkelas, M., Lange, L. O., & Halfon, N. (2003). Childbirth education classes: Sociodemographic disparities in attendance and the association of attendance with breastfeeding initiation. *Maternal and Child Health Journal, 7*(2), 87-93.

Lublin, J. S. (2001, October 16). Three Microsoft alums who used career skills to follow their passion, *Wall Street Journal.* Retrieved from: http://online.wsj.com/article/SB1003175945641002400.html.

Lyndon, A., Sexton, J. B., Simpson, K. R., Rosenstein, A., Lee, K. A., & Wachter, R. M. (2011). Predictors of likelihood of speaking up about safety concerns in labour and delivery. *BMJ Quality & Safety, 21*, 791-799. doi: 10.1136/bmjqs.2010.050211

MacDorman, M., Declercq, E., & Mathews, T. J. (2013). *Who are the women giving birth in various settings?* Paper presented at the Institute of Medicine and National Research Council Workshop on Research Issues in the Assessment of Birth Settings, Washington, D.C. Retrieved from:http://www.iom.edu/~/media/Files/Activity Files/Women/BirthSettings/6-MAR-2013/MacDorman.pdf

Main, E. K., Morton, C. H., Hopkins, D., Giuliani, G., Melsop, K., & Gould, J. B. (2011). *Cesarean deliveries, outcomes, and opportunities for change in California: Toward a public agenda for maternity care safety and quality. CMQCC White Papers.* Palo Alto, CA: California Maternal Quality Care Collaborative.

Main, E. K., Oshiro, B., Chagolla, B., Bingham, D., Dang-Kilduff, L., & Kowalewski, L. (2010). Elimination of non-medically indicated (elective) deliveries before 39 weeks gestational age. In California Department of Public

Health (Ed.), *California Toolkit to Transform Maternity Care.* Sacramento: California Department of Public Health.

Mander, R. (2001). *Supportive care and midwifery.* Osney Mead, Oxford, UK: Blackwell Science Ltd.

Manning-Orenstein, G. (1998). A birth intervention: The therapeutic effects of doula support versus Lamaze preparation on first-time mothers' working models of caregiving. *Alternative Therapies in Health and Medicine, 4*(4), 73-81.

Mardorossian, C. M. (2003). Laboring women, coaching men: Masculinity and childbirth education in the contemporary United States. *Hypatia, 18*(3), 113-134.

Martin, E. (1992). *The woman in the body: A cultural analysis of reproduction.* Boston: Beacon Press.

McMahon, M. (1995). *Engendering motherhood: Identity and self-transformation in women's lives.* New York: Guilford Press.

McNiven, P., Hodnett, E. D., & O'Brien-Pallas, L. L. (1992). Supporting women in labor: A work-sampling study of the activities of intrapartum nurses. *Birth, 19*(1), 3-9.

Michie, H., & Cahn, N. R. (1997). *Confinements: Fertility and infertility in contemporary culture.* New Brunswick, NJ: Rutgers University Press.

Monto, M. (1997). The lingering presence of medical definitions among women committed to natural childbirth. *Journal of Contemporary Ethnography, 26*(3), 293-316.

Morgen, S. (2002). *Into our own hands: The women's health movement in the United States, 1969-1990.* New Brunswick, NJ: Rutgers University Press.

Morris, T. (2013). *Cut it out: The C-section epidemic in America*. New York: New York University Press.

Morton, C. H. (2009). Where are the ethnographies of U.S. hospital births? *Anthropology News, March*, 10-11.

Morton, C. H., & Basile, M. (2013). *Medicaid coverage for doula care: Re-examining the arguments through a reproductive justice lens*. Retrieved from: http://www.scienceandsensibility.org

Morton, C. H., & Hsu, C. (2007). Contemporary dilemmas in American childbirth education: Findings from a comparative ethnographic study. *The Journal of Perinatal Education, 16*(4), 25-37. doi: 10.1624/105812407X245614

Murphy-Lawless, J. (1999). *Reading birth and death: A history of obstetrics thinking*. Indianapolis, IN: Indiana University Press.

Namey, E. E., & Lyerly, A. D. (2010). The meaning of "control" for childbearing women in the U.S. *Social Science and Medicine, 71*, 769-776.

Norman, B. M., & Rothman, B. K. (2007). The new arrival: Labor doulas and the fragmentation of midwifery and caregiving. In W. Simonds, B. K. Rothman, & B. M. Norman (Eds.), *Laboring on: Birth in transition in the United States*. New York: Routledge.

O'Brien, M. (1981). *The politics of reproduction*. Boston: Routledge and Kegan Paul.

Oakley, A. (1979). *Becoming a mother*. New York: Schocken Books.

Oakley, A. (1980). *Women confined: Toward a sociology of childbirth*. New York: Schocken Books.

Oakley, A. (1984). *The captured womb: A history of the medical care of pregnant women*. Oxford, UK: Basil Blackwell.

Oakley, A. (1993). *Essays on women, medicine, and health*. Edinburgh, UK: Edinburgh University Press.

Odent, M. (1984). *Birth reborn*. New York: Pantheon Books.

Oshiro, B., Henry, E., Wilson, J., Branch, D., & Varner, M. (2009). Decreasing elective deliveries before 39 weeks of gestation in an integrated health care system. *Obstetrics & Gynecology, 113*(4), 804-811.

Papagni, K., & Buckner, E. (2006). Doula support and attitudes of intrapartum nurses: A qualitative study from the patient's perspective. *The Journal of Perinatal Education, 15*(1), 11-18. doi: 10.1624/105812406X92949

Paterno, M. T., Van Zandt, S. E., Murphy, J., & Jordan, E. T. (2012). Evaluation of a student-nurse doula program: An analysis of doula interventions and their impact on labor analgesia and cesarean birth. *Journal of Midwifery & Women's Health, 57*(1), 28-34. doi: 10.1111/j.1542-2011.2011.00091.x

Payant, L., Davies, B., Graham, I. D., Peterson, W. E., & Clinch, J. (2008). Nurses' intentions to provide continuous labor support to women. *Journal of Obstetric, Gynecologic, and Neonatal Nursing, 37*(4), 405-414. doi: 10.1111/j.1552-6909.2008.00257.x

Perez, M. Z. (2012). *The radical doula guide: A political primer for full spectrum pregnancy and childbirth support*. Publisher: M.Z. Perez.

Perez, P. (1990/1994). *Special women: The role of the professional labor assistant.* Seattle, WA: Pennypress, Inc.

Perinatal Advisory Council. (2010). *Three things nurse wish you know about childbirth.* Retrieved from: http://www.pregnancy.org/article/three-things-nurses-wish-you-knew-about-childbirth

Perkins, B. B. (2003). *The medical delivery business: Health reform, childbirth, and the economic order.* New Brunswick, NJ: Rutgers University Press.

Pincus, J. (2000). Childbirth advice literature as it relates to two childbearing ideologies. *Birth, 27*(3), 209-213.

Placksin, S. (1994). *Mothering the new mother: Your postpartum resource companion.* New York: Newmarket Press.

Plante, L. A. (2009). Mommy, What did you do in the Industrial Revolution? Meditations on the rising Cesarean rate. *The International Journal of Feminist Approaches to Bioethics, 2,* 140-147.

Pollner, M., & Emerson, R. M. (2001). Ethnomethodology and ethnography. In P. Atkinson, A. Coffey, S. Delamont, J. Lofland, & L. Lofland (Eds.), *Handbook of ethnography* (pp. 118-135). London: Sage Publications.

Pollock, D. (1999). *Telling bodies, performing birth: Everyday narratives of childbirth.* New York: Columbia University Press.

Purdy, L. M. (1996). *Reproducing persons: Issues in feminist bioethics.* Ithaca, NY: Cornell University Press.

Raphael, D. (1973). *The tender gift: Breastfeeding.* New York: Schocken Books.

Rattner, D., Abreu, I., Araujo, M., & Santos, A. (2009). Humanizing childbirth to reduce maternal and neonatal mortality: A national effort in Brazil. In R. E. Davis-Floyd, L. M. Barclay, B. Daviss, & J. Tritten (Eds.), *Birth models that work* (pp. 385-414). Berkeley, CA: University of California Press.

Rayburn, W. F. (2011). *The obstetrician/gynecologist workforce in the United States: Facts, figures, and implications.* Washington, D.C.: American College of Obstetricians and Gynecologists.

Reed, R. K. (2005). *Birthing fathers: The transformation of men in American rites of birth.* New Brunswick, NJ: Rutgers University Press.

Regan, M., & Liaschenko, J. (2007). In the mind of the beholder: Hypothesized effect of intrapartum nurses' cognitive frames of childbirth cesarean section rates. *Qualitative Health Research, 17*(5), 612-624. doi: 10.1177/1049732307301610

Reiger, K. (2001). *Our bodies, our babies: The forgotten women's movement.* Carlton South, Victoria: Melbourne University Press.

Reiger, K., & Morton, C. H. (2012). Standardising or individualising?: A critical analysis of the 'discursive imaginaries' shaping maternity care reform. *International Journal of Childbirth, 2*(3), 173-186.

Reverby, S. M. (1987). *Ordered to care: The dilemma of American nursing, 1850-1945.* Cambridge, UK: Cambridge University Press.

Rich, A. (1995). *Of woman born: Motherhood as institution and experience.* New York: W.W. Norton.

Richards, M. P. M. (1992). Doulas and the quality of maternity services. *Birth, 19*(1), 40-41.

Romalis, S. (1981). *Childbirth: Alternatives to medical control.* Austin, TX: University of Texas Press.

Rooks, J. P. (1997). *Midwifery and childbirth in America.* Philadelphia: Temple University Press.

Roth, L., & Henley, M. (2012). Unequal motherhood: Racial-ethnic and socioeconomic disparities in cesarean sections in the United States. *Social Problems, 59*(2), 207–227.

Rothman, B. K. (1982/1991). *In labor: Women and power in the birthplace.* New York: Norton.

Sakala, C. (2010). U.S. health care reform legislation offers major new gains to childbearing women and newborns. *Birth, 37*, 337-340.

Sakala, C., & Corry, M. P. (2008). *Evidence-based maternity care: What it is and what it can achieve.* New York: Milbank Memorial Fund.

Sandelowski, M. (1984). *Pain, pleasure and American childbirth: From the twilight sleep to the Read method, 1914-1960.* Westport, CT: Greenwood Press.

Sandelowski, M. (2000). *Devices and desires: Gender, technology and American nursing.* Chapel Hill, NC: University of North Carolina Press.

Scholten, C. M. (1985). *Childbearing in American society: 1650-1850.* New York: New York University Press.

Scully, D. (1980). *Men who control women's health: The miseducation of obstetrician-gynecologists.* Boston: Houghton Mifflin.

Setubal, M. S. (2001). *The labor support course at the Seattle Midwifery School: A program evaluation.* MPH thesis, University of Washington, Seattle.

Shaw, N. S. (1974). *Forced labor: Maternity care in the United States.* New York: Pergamon.

Shearer, M. H. (1989). Commentary: When the *monitrice* is an outsider. *Birth, 16*(4), 183-184.

Shorter, E. (1991). *Women's bodies: A social history of women's encounter with health, ill-health, and medicine.* New Brunswick, NJ: Transaction Publishers.

Simkin, P. (1991). Just another day in a woman's life? Women's long-term perceptions of their first birth experience. Part I. *Birth, 18*(4), 203-210.

Simkin, P. (1992a). Just another day in a woman's life? Part II: Nature and consistency of women's long-term memories of their first birth experience. *Birth, 19*(2), 64-81.

Simkin, P. (1992b). The labor support person: Latest addition to the maternity care team. *ICEA Review, 16*(1), 1-9.

Simkin, P. (1997). What kind of advocate are you? Baby? Birth? Woman? [Instructional handout].

Simkin, P. (Date unavailable). Basic needs of childbearing women (per Maslow's hierarchy of needs). [Instructional handout].

Simkin, P., & Klaus, P. H. (2004). *When survivors give birth: Understanding and healing the effects of early sexual abuse on childbearing women.* Seattle: Classic Day Publishing.

Simonds, W., Rothman, B. K., & Norman, B. M. (2006). *Laboring on: Birth in transition in the United States.* New York: Routledge.

Sleutel, M. R. (2000). Intrapartum nursing care: A case study of supportive interventions and ethical conflicts. *Birth, 27(1)*, 38-45.

Smith, D. (1987). *The everyday world as problematic: A feminist sociology.* Boston: Northeastern University Press.

Sosa, R., Kennell, J. H., Robertson, S., & Urrutia, J. (1980). The effect of a supportive companion on perinatal problems, length of labor and mother-infant interaction. *New England Journal of Medicine, 303*, 597-600.

Sperlich, M., & Seng, J. S. (2008). *Survivor moms: Women's stories of birthing, mothering, and healing after sexual abuse.* Eugene, OR: Motherbaby Press.

Starr, P. (1982). *The social transformation of American medicine.* New York: Basic Books.

Strong, W. H. (2000). *Expecting trouble: The myth of prenatal care in America.* New York: New York University Press.

Sullivan, D. A., & Weitz, R. (1988). *Labor pains: Modern midwives and home birth.* New Haven, CT: Yale University Press.

Tew, M. (1998). *Safer childbirth? A critical history of maternity care.* New York: Free Association Books, Ltd.

The Joint Commission. (2010). *Preventing maternal death.* Sentinal Event Alert. Issue 44 Retrieved from: http://ww.jointcommission.org/sentinal_event_alert_issue_44_preventing_maternal_death

The Joint Commission. (2011). *Specifications Manual for Joint Commission National Quality Measures (v2011A): PC-02 NTSV Cesarean Section.* Retrieved from: http://manual.jointcommission.org/releases/TJC2011A/MIF0167.html

Torres, J. M. (2013). Breast milk and labour support: Lactation consultants' and doulas' strategies for navigating the medical context of maternity care. *Sociology of Health and Illness*. doi: 10.1111/1467-9566.12010

Treichler, P. (1990). Feminism, medicine and the meaning of childbirth. In M. Jacobus, E. F. Keller, & S. Shuttleworth (Eds.), *Body/Politics, women and the discourses of science* (pp. 113-138). New York and London: Routledge.

Trevathan, W. R. (1987). *Human birth: An evolutionary perspective*. New York: Aldine de Gruyter.

Tucker, A. (1999/2000). Dealing with doula doubt. *PALS Ppers: A Quarterly Publication of the Pacific Association for Labor Support*, Winter.

Tumblin, A., & Simkin, P. (2001). Pregnant women's perceptions of their nurse's role during labor and delivery. *Birth, 28*(1), 52-56.

Uttal, L., & Tuominen, M. (1999). Tenuous relationships: Exploitation, emotion and racial ethnic significance in paid child care work. *Gender and Society, 13*, 758-780.

van Teijlingen, E. (2005). A critical analysis of the medical model as used in the study of pregnancy and childbirth. *Sociological Research Online, 10*(2).

Veigaa, M. B., Lama, M., Gemeinhardta, C., Houlihanb, E., Fitzsimmons, B. P., & Hodgson, Z. G. (2011). Social support in the post-abortion recovery room: Evidence from patients, support persons and nurses in a Vancouver clinic. *Contraception, 83*, 268-273.

Walzer, S. (1998). *Thinking about the baby: Gender and transitions to parenthood*. Philadelphia, PA: Temple University Press.

Ward, J. D. (2000). *La Leche League: At the crossroads of medicine, feminism and religion.* Chapel Hill, NC: The University of North Carolina Press.

Webber, S. (2012). *The gentle art of newborn family care: A guide for postpartum doulas and caregivers.* Amarillo, TX: Praeclarus Press.

Wertz, R. W., & Wertz, D. C. (1977). *Lying-In: A history of childbirth in America.* New York: The Free Press.

Witz, A. (1992). *Professions and patriarchy.* London: Routledge.

Wolf, J. H. (2009). *Deliver me from pain: Anesthesia and birth in America.* Baltimore, MD: The Johns Hopkins University Press.

Wolf, N. (2001). *Misconceptions: Truth, lies and the unexpected on the journey to motherhood.* New York: Doubleday.

KEY INFORMANT INTERVIEWS

Arms, S. (personal communication, May 3, 2002)
Barbour, J. (personal communication, April 27, 2002).
Batacan, J. (personal communication, October 31, 2012).
Goer, H. (personal communication, January 3, 2002)
Jackson, M. (personal communication, January 23, 2002).
Lowe, C. (personal communication, January 24, 2002).
Porter, J. (personal communication, January 23, 2002).
Simkin, P. (personal communication, February 15, 2000).
Weiss, R. E. (personal communication, January 27, 2002).
Young, D. (personal communication, December 12, 2001).

Index

Association of Women's Health, Obstetric, & Neonatal Nurses (AWHONN) 224, 257–256
Australia, childbirth advocacy in 279

B

baby advocates 137–138, 140–141
backstage negotiations 235–237
back-up doula partner 160
Barbour, Joan 80
Batacan, Jeanne 257–258
Beck, Cheryl Tatano 282
Becoming a Childbirth Assistant: The Lowe Method (Lowe) 82
biases, assessment of 137, 195
Bingham, Debra 257
birth advocates 138
birth attendance, for certification 111
birth experiences
    doulas' initial 200–201
    effect of sexual abuse history on 153–154
    effect on self identity 152–153
    reframing. *See* reframing the birth experience
    traumatic 150–151, 153–154
Birthing from Within 96
Birthing from Within (England) 177–178, 290
birth junkies 201
birth memories 126–129, 324–325. *See also* reframing the birth experience
The Birth Partner (Simkin) 90
The Birth Place 34, 80–82, 95
birth plan 224
    adhering to 225, 233
    enlisting clinicians as team players 241–242
birth satisfaction, factors associated with 126–127
birth stories 39–41, 92–93, 251–252, 323–324
Birth Support Providers International 84
BirthWorks 94, 96
blogs 97
bonding theory 65, 72–74, 125, 127–128, 141, 171
    feminist critiques of 77–79, 284
Brazilian Network for the Humanization of Childbirth 293
breastfeeding counselors 277
The Business of Being Born (documentary) 31

C

California Department of Public Health 257–256
career changes 112–113
career doulas 114–115
certification 111, 148–149, 169–170

P

Pacific Association for Labor Support (PALS) 90, 91, 197, 327, 329
Painless Childbirth (Lamaze) 67
pain medication use. *See also* pain relief
  effects of doula presence on 76
  unwanted 240
pain relief
  19th century campaigns for 120
  epidurals 76, 173
  saddle block 151
  spinal anesthetics 65
  Twilight Sleep 59, 65, 120
ParentsPlace/iVillage.com 328
passive patient role 218
patient advocacy groups 237
patient advocate 75–76
Perez, Paulina (Polly) 85, 86–88, 91
personal stories of mothers 218
physical side effects
  reframing 143
physical support
  nurses and 176
physician-attended births. *See also* obstetrics
  shift from midwife-attended births 56–58
Pollner, Melvin 324
Pollock, Della 39–40
postpartum doula care 33, 179–180, 183–185, 251–252, 277
posttraumatic stress disorder 284
practice models 35–36
prenatal technologies 279
"prepared childbirth" 70
Principles and Practices of Natural Childbirth (Dick-Read) 62–63
professional labor assistants 87
professional status of doulas 169–170, 204
psychoprophylaxis 66–67. *See also* Lamaze method
psychosomatic medicine 60, 64
pushing 143, 146

R

race/ethnicity
  and community-based doula programs 287–288
  reducing disparities in childbirth outcomes 293
Raphael, Dana 33, 76, 83
reduced fees for service 205–207
reformed childbirth support (1960s-1980s) 65–74
  challenges to reform efforts 66
  emotional experience in 68–74

S

V

W

Y

CPSIA information can be obtained at www.ICGtesting.com
Printed in the USA
LVOW05s1710300914

406587LV00008B/329/P